T0187135

For the Love of Animals

For the Love of Animals

Stories from my life as a vet

Dr James Greenwood

SEVEN DIALS

First published in Great Britain in 2023 by Seven Dials,
an imprint of The Orion Publishing Group Ltd
Carmelite House, 50 Victoria Embankment
London EC4Y 0DZ

An Hachette UK Company

1 3 5 7 9 10 8 6 4 2

A CIP catalogue record for this book is
available from the British Library.

ISBN (Hardback) 978 1 3996 0552 6
ISBN (eBook) 978 1 3996 0554 0
ISBN (Audio) 978 1 3996 0555 7

Typeset by Input Data Services Ltd, Bridgwater, Somerset

Printed and bound in Great Britain by Clays Ltd, Elcograf S.p.A.

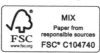

MIX
Paper from
responsible sources
FSC
www.fsc.org
FSC® C104740

www.orionbooks.co.uk

For Oliver:

Sadly, only a few months after the photograph was taken for the front cover of this book, our golden Labrador Oliver suddenly passed away just one month before his thirteenth birthday. The grief we felt is like no other but his memory will live on always and forever. As will his name, a name that we hold so dear to our hearts. This will continue to be lovingly heard in our home, as Mark and I were thrilled to welcome our first son, Oliver James, into the world just a week before this book went to print in May 2023.

This is as much Oliver's story as it is mine and it feels only right to honour his legacy in this way.

To our most handsome boy, Oliver, this book is for you. xx

CONTENTS

AUTHOR'S NOTE

This is the story of my early years as a veterinary surgeon. I've written it to share my truthful experience in a way that brings a real insight into my life as a vet and to offer you, the reader, a behind-the-scenes glimpse into the world of veterinary medicine.

A word to past and present clients and colleagues, though. If anyone believes they recognise themselves in this book, you are not recognising your *own* self. Other than friends and family, none of the characters (human or animal) are depicting any *one* individual. Every character is an amalgamation of the many interactions and experiences I've had, having spent over fifteen years working with hundreds (if not thousands) of humans and their pets. Having said that, the scenes depicted did all happen.

Furthermore, please do not take any medical or veterinary advice from the words written on these pages. I have summarised clinical proceedings to fit the narrative, so they must not be considered in any way as a reference text for veterinary medicine. If you ever have any concerns over your pet's health, please always contact your own vet immediately.

You will notice I have used the term pet 'owner' throughout. I am fully aware this phrase does not align with how the vast majority of us feel about our pets. 'Owner' suggests an animal can be likened to an inanimate object, which of course is completely preposterous. Many now prefer 'pet guardian', 'friend', 'pet parent' or 'caregiver' as more suitable turns of phrase. But, purely for the interest of simplicity, I have kept the term 'owner' in this narrative, as I believe it is still the term most people recognise to mean the person responsible for that individual animal's health and wellbeing.

Finally, a note of warning to all readers:

I have written this book true to my own experience and therefore within these pages I speak of topics and use language that some may feel is not suitable for all to read. I have shared my experience around mental health which includes a reference to suicide. It also contains descriptions of severe animal cruelty and abuse that some may find distressing. I have included resources at the end of this book (page 278) for anyone who may feel affected by any of the topics discussed.

Oliver, Part I

N. Somerset, 2010

Oliver, our one-eyed Labrador, came everywhere with us, including our tired, local pub that smelled of wet dogs, vinegar and spilled beer.

I prised a flake of white fish from its golden batter with my fork, pushed it to one side of the plate, then with my fingers sneakily offered it to the hopeful-looking canine companion sitting patiently by my side.

'You little . . .' Mark stopped himself short from across the table. 'If I'd have done that, you'd have absolutely killed me!' he said, smiling, with an astonished look of injustice.

I laughed.

'I know,' I smirked, 'but I'm allowed to, I'm his vet!' We both shared a laugh at my blatant, unashamed hypocrisy.

A Wednesday night and neither Mark nor myself could be bothered to cook, after I'd had yet another manic day in the world of veterinary medicine. I'd met Mark a few years previously. We talked online for months, penpals at first. He had been living in France, I had just moved back from Jersey, then within weeks of meeting in person we moved in together and relocated to the outskirts of Bristol.

I tucked into the artery-clogging plate of fish and chips and the mound of army-green mushy peas that had been piled on the side. The whole plate of food looked like it had been fished out from the bottom of a pond.

'Are we all done here, gents?' the waitress called, as I scraped the remnants of batter and green sludge to one side of my plate and put my cutlery down. As she came over and lifted both our plates from the table, Oliver looked up at her with his mouth wide open, the corners of his lips pulled back with anticipation and his one eye brimming with excitement. He offered this trademark cheeky, winking smile whenever he sensed there may be some food on offer.

'I 'avent got any left, darling.' The waitress spoke with a kind West Country accent directly to Oliver. 'You've eaten the last one!' The pub usually had a well-stocked kilner jar of dog biscuits on the bar, although that evening only a few crumbs remained. We thanked her, partly for the food, but mostly on Oliver's behalf for all the treats.

With the table cleared, I sat back in the chair and ran my hands down the back of my neck, pushing my fingertips into the strap of rock-hard muscle that ran down either side of my cervical spine. I massaged the knots with a circular motion until the skin on my neck had turned cherry red. For a small moment, the tension of another busy day in practice was relieved.

Unusually, Oliver was not the only dog with us that evening. We were also dog-sitting one of the veterinary nurses' dogs called Jenson. Sarah, the nurse, had been treated to a long weekend in Ireland. And this was our first night looking after him. We finished up, paid, then to give the dogs a bit of a leg stretch, took the long route back home through the village.

From the first time they met, Oliver and Jenson immediately hit it off. Jenson put the 'spring' in springer spaniel and was named after the famous racing driver. Both of a similar age, similar size and with similar levels of energy, the two young dogs loved nothing more than to run at full speed with their heads locked together like two sharks in battle. Eventually, one of them would surrender, they'd both collapse in a heap, allow themselves to catch a quick breather before one of them would inevitably entice the other and they'd both explode off around the field once again. Two wonderfully compatible canine friends.

As we walked through the churchyard, we paused to take a seat on one of the wooden benches. I hiccupped an oily reminder of the unhealthy food I'd guzzled and wished I'd chosen something more wholesome from the plastic-coated, yellow pages of the pub menu. I threw my head back and stared up into the night sky. The clean, cold evening air filled my lungs as I inhaled deeply and once again allowed the stresses of the day to escape my tense neck muscles. Oliver looked up at me with his single eye and a gentle head tilt that displayed disappointment and confusion as to why we had stopped. Ruled by his stomach, as all Labradors are, he knew the routine: the sooner we got home, the sooner he'd be enjoying his last small snack before bed.

'C'mon then, let's get you home!' I said as Mark and I heaved ourselves away from the respite of the church bench to mark the end of the evening's fayre. Oliver started to jump around, realising his staring tactics had somehow miraculously worked. I could read him like a book, yet despite that, he still had us both wrapped around his little paw.

As we reached the front door, the excitement to be off his lead meant Oliver bypassed the recollection of his evening snack and instead started running multiple laps of the downstairs living room. Jenson soon followed and then the two of them bounced in turn at the uPVC door that opened onto an enclosed patio area.

Neither the indoor lounge nor outdoor patio were quite big enough for them to run at full pace, but it was large enough that Oliver could perform some pretty nimble figure of eights, zooming between the living room and the outside patio, navigating the narrow doorway with surprising accuracy given his cycloptic, single-vision perspective. Jenson followed only centimetres behind. Eventually, though, the zoomies dissipated and they both settled. We closed the doors and left them downstairs. I sprinkled a few treats over each of their beds and then dragged my own weary body upstairs.

Knowing that I had another overbooked day of consults to follow, I set my alarm, switched the lights off and closed my eyes.

I slept so very deeply that night. The kind of sleep that when you wake, it seems impossible to tell if you've been asleep for five minutes or five hours.

This time, it was the latter. But something didn't feel quite right. An unfamiliar ringtone screamed, loud and obnoxious. I didn't recognise the tune. Not my alarm. Not Mark's alarm. I slowly regained consciousness and looked over the edge of the bed for my phone. I tapped the LED screen. The brightness bleached my eyes as I looked away and then back again.

It was 5.03 a.m.

My mind was racing as I tried to kickstart my brain into function.

The ringing continued.

I looked across to the other side of the bed to see Mark's phone had sprung to life. Shining brightly, flashing on and off, vibrating along the bedside table, shuffling dangerously towards the edge.

I nudged him in the back to wake him up.

'It's your phone,' I said, half asleep. 'Someone's ringing you.'

Annoyed, I rolled back to my side of the bed, covered my eyes with the fold of my elbow to block out the dawn sunlight and hoped I might drift off for another couple of hours of kip before the new day *officially* started.

Sleepily, he answered. 'Hello?' There was a pause. 'Yeah, that's me.'

I remained still but continued to listen in.

I felt the bed agitate as Mark started to lift himself up into a sitting position, and shuffled to lean his back against the bedhead. I could sense an urgency in the way he moved as he pulled the pillow from behind his waist and threw it on the bedroom floor.

I looked over at him and mouthed, 'Who is it?' I hoped he might return a silent clue. A cold caller perhaps, or someone from the international language school he worked at. Something that meant I could go back to sleep. Fingers crossed.

Instead, he shook his head at me and held out his hand as if to say, 'not now, hang on'.

He pushed back the duvet and stepped out of bed. With

the handset still pressed against his head, he walked towards the window.

'No, it can't be, he's downstairs in the kitchen,' I heard him say.

By then, I too was wide awake and upright in the bed, engrossed and captivated by the conversation as it played out.

For someone usually so positive and bright, there was an uncharacteristic seriousness to Mark's tone. He then lowered the handset into the palm of his hand and hit the speakerphone button.

Midway through a sentence, and through the muffled fuzzy quality of the phone's built-in speakers, a woman's voice echoed around the bedroom: 'Opposite side of his one eye . . . I just came round the corner and he's here. I'm on the main road and got your number from the tag on his collar . . .'

I looked again to Mark, whose face had melted into frowned confusion.

'What's happened?' I mouthed.

'She says she has Oliver,' he whispered back quietly.

'WHAT?' I said in disbelief.

'Hang on, just listen,' he signalled back, not wanting the stranger on the line to overhear that we were talking without her.

'It can't be,' I whispered calmly.

Suddenly the voice from the phone echoed once again. 'I've pulled over and I'll stay with him. Are you nearby?'

I looked at Mark and he stared back at me. Before we had a chance to answer, the voice continued. 'I'm not sure what's happened, but I think you should come pretty quickly,' she said shakily. 'He is alive . . . but I think he's been hurt.'

WHAT? We looked at each other in total bewilderment as her words echoed around the room.

A high-pitched yelp suddenly sounded through the telephone handset; it was a dog's yelp. A dog in distress. I recognised the sound immediately. I knew it was Oliver, but my brain wouldn't allow me to believe it. My heart sank. I threw my hand to my mouth and stared at Mark. His face transitioned from confusion to utter panic.

'It's OK, it's OK,' the voice said, trying to calm and reassure the dog lying beside her. 'I think . . . I think he's been hit by a car.'

My heart rate quickened and I leapt out of bed. I rushed round to the other side of the room, out of the bedroom door and down the stairs as quickly as I could, taking two or three steps at a time, and holding on to the banister as I flew.

Mark was already leaning forwards, his head pressed against the glass pane of the bedroom window and his neck angled at ninety degrees, trying to visualise the front of the house.

'I can't see anything!' he shouted from upstairs.

Then, suddenly, everything fell into place. My feet were frozen on the spot as I stood with my hands on my head, shaking in disbelief as I reached the bottom of the stairs to find our front door was wide open, swinging forwards and backwards in the early morning breeze.

'They've gone!' I yelled back.

Both Oliver and Jenson were nowhere to be seen.

CHAPTER 1

Bertie

Huddersfield, West Yorkshire, 1990

'Aaaaaaagh!' I heard my mother shriek from outside my bedroom.

I pretended not to hear her. The warm hug from my giraffe-print duvet was too cosy and comfy for me to care about anything else so early in the morning.

'Where is he?' My mother's voice echoed along the landing. 'JAMES?' she called out.

I rubbed the crystals of sleep from the corners of my eyes and looked at the Wallace and Gromit alarm clock beside my bed. It was 7 a.m. The school bus wasn't for at least another hour but, for some reason, that morning, a sense of urgency had descended on the morning family routine.

In our house, with most things, there was often an initial descent into drama, but I kinda knew that if I kept my nose out and left everyone to their own devices, things usually settled down with a bit of time. So I rolled over and waited for the storm to pass. This time, though, I was wrong. I squeezed open my eyes to find the silhouette of my mother standing at my bedroom door. She wore a cream-coloured dressing gown and looked rather pale despite her olive complexion. With one hand on her hip, her other arm was raised out to her side and her index finger pointed to something down the corridor.

'Get up and get out here NOW!' Each stern word was forced out with a strict maternal discipline. Her hand was trembling. I could sense trouble was brewing.

I flung back my patterned duvet and followed her out. My dad and older sister were already waiting on the landing. The four of us gathered into a circle and stared down at our feet, each wondering what on earth it was that we were witnessing.

In the dead of night, a mysterious creature had somehow deposited itself in the middle of our landing carpet. It had a brown, elongated, smooth body shaped like a curled-up Cumberland sausage, and from the centre, at what I guessed was the head end, sprang several long tentacles.

'What is it?' my teenage sister asked.

I knelt to the ground and leant forwards, slowly lowering my head to take a closer look. With only about a foot between the creature and the tip of my nose, I rubbed both my eyes. I squinted to see without my glasses on, but I could just about make out that the creature had gills. And fins. And it kind of looked like it was upside down.

Then, suddenly . . . it moved. All four of us jumped. With lightning speed, the creature unravelled itself counter clockwise and then recoiled in the opposite direction.

At that point, my sister screamed. 'BLAAAAAAAGH!'

'Oh, Nicola!' my mother retorted.

My dad lifted his foot, removed his slipper and raised it high above his head ready to dispatch of this uninvited guest.

'STOP!' I shouted.

I pushed my face even closer, feeling a desperate responsibility to solve this enigma. Animals were, after all, my department. And then, it dawned on me. It was Bertie! Bertie was an eel-shaped fish called a weather loach who had quite happily (until that morning) lived his life lurking in the gravelled base of my bedroom aquarium.

It turns out, unbeknown to me at the time, that weather loaches are called such as they are able to predict changes in atmospheric pressure, leaping from drought-threatened habitats in search of somewhere more favourable; a fish able to survive for several hours out of water by gulping down great mouthfuls of air, extracting the oxygen, and releasing the rest in small bouts of fishy flatulence. Quite fascinating stuff and, true to nature, Bertie had attempted this daredevil stunt himself.

However, rather than discovering new exciting territories, marshes, bogs or mangroves, he found himself instead at seven o'clock in the morning on our landing carpet, having narrowly missed being trodden on by my half-asleep, barefoot and very disgruntled mother on her way to start the breakfast. I quickly scooped him up and carried him in my cupped hands down the hallway into my bedroom and lowered him gently back into the cool water. Miraculously, he survived, forever more trapped in his tank by the pile of *Practical Fishkeeping* magazines I had collected over the years now weighted on the aquarium hood (Mother's request).

Growing up, there was not a day that went by without me hearing the word 'JAMES' being yelled, or shrieks, gasps or cries for 'HELP!' as my animal family crossed paths with my human family. In hindsight, the reaction of my poor long-suffering mother wasn't entirely unjustified as this wasn't the first, or last, time something like this happened. Wherever animals are involved, in whatever capacity, you can always expect the unexpected. And my later childhood, especially, was full of animals.

I wasn't raised on a farm, or even in the countryside. Instead, I grew up on the outskirts of Huddersfield town centre. Rows of houses with neat lawns, soot-scarred stonework and a friendly community spirit – the typical warmth of Yorkshire suburbia where you could knock on a friend's door at any time of day and end up staying for tea. I had a comfortable upbringing. We definitely weren't spoilt as children, but I also don't really recall any troubles. All I could decipher of my own father's career was that he was a 'businessman' and went to 'business meetings'.

I always looked at my father and thought it seemed boring at the time, dressing up in a suit and going to work. Too much like school. Although I can now, with hindsight, recognise just how incredibly hard he worked for his family. Weekdays were spent in the office and even when he got home, his briefcase overflowed with paperwork and documents well into the evenings. Then, most weekends, my parents would get dressed up and attend one of the many corporate dinners – my dad in a tuxedo, Mum often in a silk floral dress, huge eighties shoulder pads and a pair of large clip-on diamond earrings that made her earlobes hurt. Saturday night was the night my sister and I were allowed to stay up and watch *Blind Date*. There was something I loved about the sickly sweet smell of the twenty-pence bag of sweets balanced on my lap, mixed with the volatile aroma of hairspray and Chanel perfume that accompanied my mother as she swished up to us in the lounge and placed a kiss on both our foreheads before leaving me and my sister in the caring company of Cilla Black and a babysitter.

On the surface, there was nothing really about my two parents or the house into which I was born that would make anyone predict it'd spawn an animal-obsessed misfit like me, hell-bent on converting every corner of our home and garden into a multi-species suburban menagerie. On my mother's side, though, my great-grandpa was a medical pathologist. During the war he practised out of the family home. His main speciality was in the diagnosis, treatment and prevention of venereal disease. It might well be approached differently nowadays but, at the time, sexually transmitted diseases weren't thought to be a hugely appropriate topic to discuss with us as the young great-grandchildren of this liberal, forward-thinking physician – mainly to avoid the inevitably awkward questions around what the words 'gonorrhoea' and 'chlamydia' meant, and probably to stop us from using them in everyday conversations – *So, could I catch gonorrhoea, Gran?* I can't really claim his life as a practitioner had a huge medical influence on me growing up, as we didn't really know much about his career other than having a vague understanding that Great-Grandpa was the doctor in the family.

Perhaps more on topic, though, on my father's side, my grandma *was* raised on a farm. And this I *was* allowed to know all about. I loved her stories, really loved her stories. They transported my young impressionable mind to the hill-tops around Hebden Bridge. I pictured the horse and cart she rode to deliver fresh milk to the village, the faithful collie dog sent to round up the flock of hardy hill sheep and the day a herd of dairy cows slipped and slid down the cobbled lanes of Heptonstall one snowy winter. Her farming life completely captivated me. I absorbed every detail from her past and would ask to hear the same stories over and over, playing them out in my mind. I aspired as a young boy to one day live on a farm, encouraged by Grandma, and whenever I told her of my grand plan, she would tap her hand on my shoulder and in her thick Yorkshire dialect giggle the words, 'Aye, champion', as her official seal of approval.

And so, with medicine on one side of my family and farming on the other, perhaps it was nature that firmly planted a 'veterinary seed'. For that seed to grow, though, it still required nurture – and it was nurture that allowed my veterinary dream to flourish. Casting my mind back as far as I possibly can, even my earliest blurred childhood memory involves animals, on the hilltop sheep farm belonging to my great-aunt, high up in the bleak moorlands of the Pennine Hills. An old Yorkshire stone farmhouse with small windows and low ceilings, kept warm by an open coal fire that roared in the sitting room through the twelve months of the year – the only buffer against the ever-present grey cloud sky and driving rain outside. The porch smelled of wet dogs, wellington boots and tar from the coal smoke. The air outside, in contrast, was filled with the deliciously sweet, punchy, vinegary smell of grass silage which, to this day, is a guaranteed trigger to make my mouth water. Various stone and tin-clad outbuildings housed all sorts of exciting clutter and at the farm gate a sheepdog barked loudly, tethered to the end of a metal chain with strict instructions to all children not to approach 'unless yer want t'av yer 'ead ripped off'. It was a typically harsh hilltop farm with an unforgiving climate.

'Hard graft' is perhaps the most succinct summary, but I was captivated and loved our visits.

In the late eighties, one frosty February, I can distinctly remember the rough cracked hands of the shepherd as he gripped me by the wrist and wrapped my hand around a cold, slimy grey lump that dangled from the back end of a ewe. I can't have been more than four years old. His skin, like sandpaper, grated against my soft, squidgy Play-Doh fingers as he moulded our hands together, forming a tight grip around the lamb's foot.

'Now, PULL!' I felt him draw the leg towards us.

A rapid torrent of warm red fluid soon cascaded towards us and hit the ground. Through the biting cold air, steam rose from the dark, wet Yorkshire cobbles like the dry ice of a stage production and, as we let go, through the mist, a mysterious package had landed right by my feet. The shepherd ripped through the outer wrapping like a frenzied child playing pass the parcel and then from the pool of fluid and membranes emerged the wet head of a newborn lamb. Confused but enthralled, I heard a gentle round of congratulations erupt from the smiling group of adults that circled around me, unsure if it was for me or for the lamb. We retired back into the farmhouse for Sunday lunch and while the family continued to catch up, I sat mesmerised, with a million questions buzzing around my infant brain.

Witnessing new life is always a vivid experience but even at four years old I knew something monumental had just happened. Of course, I was far too young to understand the biology – but even now, as I write these words, I can still feel it: the same fascination, the thrill, the intrigue that flooded my soul that day. Something happened, something perhaps otherworldly. I felt an inexplicable connection, a magical adrenaline rush. Without any doubt in my mind, my own innate subconscious relationship with animals was born in that same moment, on that very day, alongside that very lamb.

I wasn't lucky enough to live on a farm, but with such formative early animal experiences, that didn't stop my attempts to bring the country life back to our home in suburbia. At the end of our road there was a patch of scrubland we, somewhat romantically, referred to as 'the secret garden'. A deserted, overgrown plot that had sat on the market for decades. Untouched, completely left to nature and a great place for a young naturalist mind to explore. I would sneak through the rotten wooden gates with my best friend, Victoria, as we trampled through the undergrowth of thick brambles and nettles in the hope of spotting some potential suburban wildlife: a den of fox cubs, hedgehogs, perhaps even a tawny owl.

Sometimes we did. But sadly, being on the outskirts of town, we had more chance of finding a few empty pop cans, discarded food containers and, on one occasion, a used condom – which we poked with sticks and laughed so uncontrollably at that we very nearly collapsed. Still, all very educational for two young minds! Our 'secret garden' obviously wasn't that much of a secret to the rest of Huddersfield, looking back now, but the wilderness it provided was a great place for uninhibited adventures.

And, in Victoria, I had a true friend as our seven-year-old worlds collided beautifully over a shared love for animals. We also loved to dress up in her mother's old clothes, watch *Eurovision* and puff on fake cigarettes, but, nevertheless, animals were always nearby. We shared a 'ciggie' nearly every time we cleaned out the guinea pigs. Great bellowing clouds of talcum powder forced from the end of white cardboard tubes that dangled from our lips as we chatted nonsense and occasionally tapped the tip of scrumpled gold foil against the roofing felt of the guinea-pig hutch. And then, once again, we would fall about laughing. And when we weren't chain-smoking, we explored the secret garden, tended to the toy farm set sprawled in my attic and recorded a weekly 'radio show' about animal rights on our ghetto blaster. With Victoria by my side my early childhood really was carefree and completely joyous.

Looking back, I probably do owe everything to animals. I also owe everything to my parents for allowing me to indulge my curiosity with animals and for their trust in me to look after them.

The general expectation of boys growing up in the early nineties, especially in Yorkshire, was that you would play sport. I tried cricket but couldn't catch. Then football but I couldn't run very fast. And as for rugby – well, I was too busy learning the words to the debut album from a new group called the Spice Girls. I was useless at all sport (causing much confusion and disappointment in our keen sporting family) so no one really knew *what* to do with me.

My parents tried everything. 'Look here, at the music!' our piano teacher would screech at me as she frantically tapped at the pages of 'Three Blind Mice' with the end of her HB pencil. I drove the poor woman to despair as I random-ly hammered down on any one of the cream-coloured keys of her expensive black shiny piano, while looking over my shoulder or down at my feet, searching for even the tiniest glimpse of her two black cats.

'The boy is too distracted. If he's not asking about the frogs in the pond then he's too obsessed with finding the cats. It's hopeless,' I overheard her report back to my mother when she came to pick me up.

With music and sport both certified non-starters, it became clear that unless animals were involved, whatever hobbies were thrust upon me just could not hold my attention.

Animals have remained a stable constant through my entire life – an influence that shaped and developed me as a person then, and still does today. Two goldfish came first (great choice), quickly followed by two unhandleable Russian dwarf hamsters (terrible choice). Two guinea pigs (not actually our choice) arrived as a surprise Christmas present from my uncle one year (his choice) and then rabbits the next (a very lovely choice).*

Meanwhile, a tortoiseshell cat called Toffee lived in the kitchen, rescued by my parents before I was born, and no matter how many times I crouched to the floor, rubbed my thumb against my first two fingers and made the infamous 'kissy lip noise' that everyone seems to do when they are being ignored by cats, I could never tempt her to stay anything less than six feet away from me. I was often on the receiving end of a mean hiss and a Tyson-inspired right hook, which is cat language for 'I-warned-you-small-human-to-get-the-hell-out-of-my-kitchen!'

After this sass-puss sadly slimmed down to a tiny waif due to her failing kidneys, she passed at a remarkable twenty years old. And so then, and only then, came the huge family

---

* FYI – as much as we loved them, I absolutely do not endorse the gifting of pets as presents to children!

decision to bring a puppy into our home. A Cavalier King Charles spaniel we called Smudge. She was our first family dog and quickly gained the adoration of us all. She had a lovely white blaze down the centre of her caramel face, with two large, doting brown eyes and long floppy ears. A splodge of misplaced caramel fur smeared across the white of her muzzle (hence the name 'Smudge') which meant she was 'imperfect' according to the breed standard, but we didn't care. She was gentle and sweet-natured, and the perfect first family dog.

By the time I reached my early teen years I had crammed my bedroom with tank upon tank, which housed a whole array of residents whose names read longer than my class register: pufferfish, stick insects, tropical fish, fire-bellied salamanders, cold-water fish (including the immortal Bertie and his adrenaline-fuelled lifestyle choices), all housed along one wall, with aquatic frogs and red-clawed crabs showcased along the next, then a smaller row of tanks housed the offspring of a group of polyamorous guppy fish. Never one to be held back by the constraints of four bedroom walls, I even seized an opportunity to claim and convert the disused Wendy house in the back garden into a rather smart poultry mansion for five feather-footed bantams from Clitheroe poultry market who took up residence in the penthouse suite of nesting boxes I had attached at waist height.

Then, by about fourteen, I had honed my negotiating skills and managed to convince the gatekeepers of my small suburban zoo (i.e. my parents) that ducks would be a great idea – a 'gardener's best friend' – on the promise they would hoover up any slugs and snails. Although I hadn't quite realised how destructive the four webbed feet of a pair of ducks could be, as Molly and Daisy trampled their daily path through the neat foliage in search of sluggy snacks. 'Slug-free and flattened' wasn't quite the garden aesthetic my green-fingered parents had been promised.

The ducks, sadly, never quite managed to win over the other humans in the house – messy, smelly, loud (the ducks, that is) – and despite my repeated attempts to educate them (my family, that is), the ducks just didn't help themselves and instead seemed to bring a whole new level of feathery calamity to every situation. An encounter with a fox led to an altercation involving a broom handle and then, more specifically, on the morning of my parents' silver wedding anniversary things *really* came to a head.

'Animals bloody EVERYWHERE!' screeched my exasperated mother, both of us in our wellington boots holding brooms, her in a posh frock, as we frantically swept against a rising tsunami of floating poultry sewage. The caterers had to leap and dance around us as the tide of manure crept ever closer to the edge of the pristine white marquee, all courtesy of a burst hosepipe that had flooded the duck house – just twenty minutes before guests were due to arrive.

She was, of course, right – as mothers tend to be. There were *indeed* animals everywhere. My plan to convert the back garden of our house on our residential lane on the outskirts of town into a fully functional farmyard seemed, somehow, to be slowly working. But I still had one last idea to pitch. And it involved the secret garden.

I had started secondary school and on leaving for the school bus, I had very mysteriously asked my parents if we could talk about 'something' when I got home later that day.

'What's this all about?' my mother asked in a nervous

tone as she pulled up a chair to the kitchen table.

'No, we have to wait for Dad,' I replied, putting the brakes on.

'DAD, COME ON!' I shouted.

He left his desk of neatly arranged documents upstairs and made his way down to the kitchen.

'What's the matter?' he said as he pulled out a seat from under the table and joined my mother opposite me. He loosened his tie, folded his arms and reclined back into the rounded arc of the pine kitchen chair.

'Has something happened at school?' Mum asked reluctantly.

'No, no, nothing like that. It's just, I've been thinking for a long time now about something . . .'

A wave of uncertainty hit me mid-flow and suddenly the dialogue I had rehearsed in my head felt clumsy.

'Go on then?' My dad sat forwards from his chair, unfolded his arms and placed them on the table.

'OK. You know I've not really ever been any good at things like playing football or—'

'Rugby, golf, yes . . .' he interrupted, his two biggest passions in life in which I shared little interest.

I hesitated. Maybe this wasn't such a good idea.

'But . . . I like other things instead?' I continued.

'Right, and . . . ?' Mum said, in a kind of hurried but encouraging manner.

'OK, well . . .' I took in a deep breath before continuing. 'I think . . . we . . . or, more, I . . . because you won't have to have anything to do with this at all . . . because . . . I mean, I will do everything . . . but . . .'

The anticipation was killing them. They looked terrified

at whatever I was about to say, if I could only get my jumbled words into a formed sentence.

With one final deep breath, I decided to just come out and say it: 'I think we should get a goat.'

As soon as the words left my mouth, their faces shifted from terrified and concerned to complete confusion as the three of us sat in silence just staring at each other.

'Get . . . a goat?' my dad mirrored back at me in disbelief.

At the same time, my mother (who didn't have 'get a goat' on her list of possible conversation topics with her adolescent son) stood up. Through the screeching sound of her chair legs scraping along the kitchen floor tiles, she broke her own silence with a loud 'OH-FOR-GOODNESS-SAKE . . .' as she pulled the tea towel that was draped from over her shoulder, screwed it up and thrust it on the kitchen table.

A fantastic cook, my mother returned to the hob and gave a pot of Bolognese a good stir before she lifted the spoon to her lips and slurped a taste. Fighting through the heat and passing the sauce around her mouth, inhaling and exhaling around each word, she asked, 'How are you going to keep a poor goat in the middle of Huddersfield?!'

She had a point.

I looked back at my father, as he waited to hear my proposal.

'Well, I can walk her to graze the brambles in the secret garden, then I could fence off some of the lawn and she could sleep . . . she could sleep . . .' I hurried out the words in case there was any glimmer of hope, but he had already started to heave his tired body back out of the wooden chair and retire towards the door. I was losing hope. My pitch was a complete disaster, and my ship was sinking fast.

I pushed my chair back and followed after him, spitting my words out as fast as I could: 'She could sleep in the garage and she won't be any trouble' – I knew this was a little bit of a small lie – 'but I just really do think we really need a goat.' Now the desperation in my voice reached a fever pitch.

He paused. 'But why do we NEED a goat? No one else seems to NEED a goat!' my father continued, overemphasising the word NEED each time he said it.

I then realised I had completely overlooked the whole point of my request. 'So we can have milk,' I replied, with a furrowed brow that questioned whether that bit wasn't *obvious*.

'Milk?' he repeated, only louder, which told me that milking a goat wasn't the obvious part at all (major oversight on my part!).

'And what's next? Turn the garage into a dairy?' he continued, in complete disbelief and mockery.

Truth is, I hadn't actually thought that far ahead but when he said it, a small dairy at the back of the garage didn't half sound like a bad idea to me at all. I caught him glance across the kitchen at my mum, who replied with nothing more than a big wide stare, both eyes forced wider than their natural aperture should allow and lips clenched tightly shut as if to say, 'Sort this out!'

'I think that face says it all,' he said, throwing me a playful wink. 'You'll just have to wait till you're older.' He patted me on the back and walked out.

I turned back to my mother, but as I opened my mouth she beat me to it. 'Don't utter another word! The answer is no!' she said, smirking in shock at my preposterous proposition. 'Once you're older and you've got a place of your own, you can have as many goats, fish, dogs, chickens and cows as you want.' She switched the extractor fan on to full blast and turned the gas to high. 'You can have a hippopotamus for all I care!' Over the roaring hum of the fan motor and the popping sounds of her bubbling sauce, she pointed her index finger at me, stifling back a giggle, and shouted the words: 'But until then . . . NO . . . MORE . . . ANIMALS!'

CHAPTER 2

Hank

I reached secondary school well before the days when mobile phones were commonplace. The only option to make a phone call was to use the public payphone situated in the corridor outside the headmaster's office. I lifted the receiver and found a grubby twenty-pence piece at the bottom of my school rucksack. I gave it a quick wipe before posting it into the metal slot of the payphone, making a guess that twenty pence should hopefully allow at least thirty seconds of talk time. I punched in the numbers and cautiously waited, hoping that someone, anyone, would answer.

After three long rings, a voice suddenly appeared on the line. 'Hello?'

'Mum, it's me. I've not got long but I need your help.'

'Why? What's happened?'

'Can you come and collect something from me at school? It's important.'

'Collect something?' she asked, confused.

'Just . . . something.'

'What do you mean, collect something? James? What's going on?'

'YOU HAVE TEN SECONDS OF TIME REMAINING,' the automated voice of the telecom service spoke over our conversation.

'I haven't got much time,' I said. 'I'll explain when you get here.'

'James, I'm not driving all the way into the middle of Bradford unless you tell me what's . . .' The line rang dead.

ARRRGH. My idea had failed. I replaced the handset, grabbed my rucksack and hurried through the crowded corridors, pushing my way through to reach my next lesson, desperately trying to think up plan B before breaktime.

During French class, our group recital of the words *'J'écoute de la musique'* was interrupted by a knock on the classroom door. The school secretary appeared.

'Ah, James, could I borrow you for a second?'

My face immediately blushed beetroot as the synchronised 'Oooooh!' erupted from the other pupils in the room. I stood and followed her out.

'I've been asked to bring you to the headmaster's office,' the school secretary said over her shoulder, as she marched along the wooden parquet floor of the school corridor. I followed a few paces behind.

The headteacher was a typically intimidating man. He seemed to purposefully tower above his pupils whenever he addressed us, and had a thickly grown moustache which amplified the sound of his nasal breathing as it whistled rhythmically down the microphone in morning assembly.

As we entered his office, he had perched himself against the huge mahogany desk with his two legs crossed over at the ankles, in a not quite sitting but not quite standing 'lean'. Without breaking his telephone conversation, he beckoned us by waggling a hooked index finger in the air as if to say 'enter'. We crossed the threshold into the wood-panelled room and the secretary heaved the large oak door closed. The whole fusty room stank of his stale coffee and tobacco breath mixed with the tannins of the cracked leather chair he had relinquished in favour of his characteristic 'desk lean'.

'Yes, he's with me now,' the headteacher said into the mouthpiece of the telephone receiver pressed to his ear. He lowered the handset to the lapel of his charcoal-grey suit in an attempt to muffle and control how much could be shared down the line and then said in a hushed voice, 'I have your mother on the phone. She has asked me to find out what it is you need her to come and collect from you?'

My heart was racing.

'Right, well . . .'

Never one able to think on my feet, I decided that honesty was the best policy. The situation was bigger than any embarrassment I might feel, and there might be a life at stake. So I reached in and gently unhooked the legs of the stowaway passenger that had been clinging all morning to the inside seam of my blazer pocket. Then I pulled out my hand and held it out in front of me. The headteacher and school secretary both leant forwards. I slowly opened my cupped palm to reveal a lime-green twig, no bigger than a matchstick, with two long antennae and six spindly legs, gently swaying from side to side.

'What the hell is that?' the headteacher asked, pulling his face into a grimace while the school secretary recoiled in horror.

'Sir,' I hesitated, 'I've been trying to breed my stick insects and . . . I think it's worked.'

The baby arthropod must have hatched in the night, crawled from the uncovered tray on my bedside table and found her way onto my blazer, which lay dumped on the floor. Only to be discovered, halfway through morning assembly, when I suddenly felt a gentle tickle on the back of my neck.

They both stared at me in silence.

'I was wondering if she might come and pick her up for me,' I tentatively muttered in a quiet voice, still with my palm outstretched. 'And, also . . . could you ask her to shut my bedroom door . . . please?'

I had suddenly realised that there must have been at least one hundred eggs scattered like poppy seeds across the uncovered sheet of moistened kitchen roll laid out on a tray under my bed. I had the nightmare vision of them exploding like popcorn into little green sticks, crawling free and migrating around the entire house.

The headteacher looked perplexed as he relayed this information back to my mother. I couldn't decipher much of the conversation as it continued to play out, but I could overhear a lot of apologising. He replaced the handset and sat down in his chair, taking his time to think through how to deliver his verdict.

'Your mother says that *thing* will survive perfectly fine in your lunchbox.'

YES! Great thinking! I thought to myself.

'BUT, let this be a formal warning, Greenwood,' he continued. 'Any more and you'll find yourself in DETENTION!'

I think it's fair to claim that my illegal (if accidental)

smuggling of a pet onto school property for an impromptu 'show and tell' in the headmaster's office counts as my first active step towards veterinary medicine, involving both my education and animals!

Animals weren't just a part of my childhood, though, they *were* my childhood. Through writing this book, I've spent a lot of time taking my mind back to those early childhood memories. How safe I felt with animals around me. I would talk to them, worry about them, and I'd want to protect them, nurture them, feed them, pet them. My animal knowledge had to be sought through books, magazines or passed down through word of mouth. It quickly became a part of my identity – that I wanted to learn as much as I could about animals.

When it came to actually making some serious decisions, though – choosing which life route I should take – it is perhaps unsurprising that getting into vet school became my sole and absolute life's ambition.

Veterinary medicine was (and still is) a largely oversubscribed course. The odds of getting in were stacked against me. A crucial step to getting a foot in the veterinary door, though, was to gain some first-hand experience 'behind the scenes' in a vet's practice. Undeterred by the slim chances of success, at fifteen I applied for a Saturday job at our local vet's surgery. A month later, before school, a handwritten note arrived through the post and, unusually, it was addressed to me.

Sutcliffe & Wells Veterinary Surgeons
Station Road
Huddersfield

25/9/1998

Dear James,

In reply to your letter of 24/8/98 with regards to voluntary work with the surgery.

After the summer there is a vacancy for work experience on a Saturday morning 8.45–12 noon.

Please can you telephone Kym Gledhill VN, the head nurse, to discuss this matter further.

Yours sincerely,

Jayne Oxley VN.

My golden ticket. This was my 'in'. Volunteering at a vet's practice might not seem that exciting to most fifteen-year-olds, but for me, the chance to go behind the scenes at a vet's felt like I'd been given a backstage pass at a concert to meet my idol. For the next three and a half years, every Saturday was spent cleaning kennels, wiping tables, feeding the patients and cleaning up after them – taking on the role of general dogsbody to observe and absorb as much veterinary insight as I possibly could.

And I loved it. Well, I think I loved it. I look back now, having spent every Saturday morning working to build and add weight to my vet school application, and wonder whether it's really that healthy or even plausible, at fifteen, to try to make plans for what to do with the rest of your life. I was perhaps blinkered by my own unwavering passion and determination and sacrificed all other interests to get into veterinary medicine – I wonder now how much I missed out on while chasing my dream.

However, the excitement I felt the first time I watched a surgical operation on a dog or shadowed a vet as she removed a wolf tooth from a horse, the adrenaline rush of helping out with a cow caesarean – I could not ignore that fire in my belly to do more, learn more, be more 'like them' and eventually become a vet myself. I knew that if I didn't at least *try* to get into vet school, then I would regret it for the rest of my life. And so, in 2001, I sent off my university application to study veterinary medicine.

When the university offer landed in the post, after all my hard work, I'm not exaggerating when I say the exhilaration I felt was the same as I imagine it would be if I won the lottery. It's sometimes easy to look back and subconsciously trivialise the significance of these milestone moments in life, but at the time, the sheer excitement was overwhelming. All my doubts, worries, the disbelief in myself, the questioning: it all completely vanished and was replaced instead with pure elation, a huge buzz, an electrifying sense of achievement and purpose. And through feeling so excited, it confirmed in my mind that veterinary medicine was *exactly* why I was put on this earth and *exactly* what I wanted to do with my life.

Vet school was everything I had hoped for and then more. It was, though, extremely hard work. The first three years were very much focused on learning the science of how a healthy animal functions; a molecular level understanding of the intricacies of physiology, pharmacology, microbiology and biochemistry. Exam after exam, after exam.

Despite the hours spent with my head in a textbook, there were (thankfully) some practical sessions to break things up. Anatomy, first taught as diagrams on paper in lecture theatres, prepared first-year vet students for the 'real deal' in the dissection suite. A row of stainless-steel tables hosted the group dissection classes, using cadavers that had died from natural causes to allow each student to build a three-dimensional spatial awareness and appreciation of the location of nerves, vessels, organs and musculature of a myriad of species. Not for the faint-hearted.

Then came animal handling – a rare opportunity to actually interact with a living creature. Students had no choice about which creature they would face each week. The first time I held a degu (a giant gerbil-like creature), the little blighter bit me. I also remember holding a royal python for the first time ever. And I'll never forget my Geordie friend Natalie (with heart set on being a feline-only specialist vet from day dot) being held hostage in the back of a pen, shouting 'haddaway n' shite' while a randy, spitting llama danced circles around her.

In addition to the endless lectures and various practical sessions of the syllabus, there was another compulsory part of the pre-clinical training that involved working through the 'holidays' on various farming establishments. Twelve compulsory weeks of free labour in the guise of 'experience' – useful, perhaps, but three months of unpaid labour often only added to the enormous student debt that was clocked up over the five years of study.

By the time I'd reached the second year of vet school, farm animal reproduction had become a large part of our syllabus – weeks spent milking cows, lambing pregnant ewes, and then eventually I headed to the outskirts of Barnsley to complete my pig placement. My very best friend Helen, who I had met at uni and clicked with immediately from day one, and I had plotted to 'buddy up' like a pair of schoolkids and complete the compulsory three weeks together.

I had never before stepped foot on a pig farm. Pigs were and are, in fact, one of my very favourite animals. Dick King-Smith (second only to Gerald Durrell) was my childhood hero. I can see the cover of his *Triffic Pig Book* in my child's mind now, as I thumbed each page over and over and studied the image of each breed of pig with immense fascination. I even remember it became a bit of a 'thing', worryingly. 'Here you go, pig boy,' one of my mum's friends once affectionately joked as she handed me a second-hand copy of *The Sheep-Pig* from her own daughter's book collection.

Pigs were just my thing – and I say this: pigs are remarkable animals. So remarkable that some behavioural experts compare their cognitive function to the intelligence of a toddler.

So, going from being 'pig boy' in my childhood to stepping foot on a pig farm in my early twenties, all in the name of education, felt both thrilling, fitting and exciting. Learning the ins and outs of intensive pig farming, though, was quite an eye-opener.

'Stay back!' the farmhand, Kate, shouted towards us. She was a feisty local lass with bottle-dyed flame-red hair and gold ear piercings. She suffered no fools.

The farm was made up of around twenty different buildings. Some were traditional stone barns, others looked more like the white corrugated buildings you might see on an industrial retail park – windowless buildings with giant air-conditioning fans encased behind black metal cages attached to the outside walls.

Kate had ordered us to stand behind some metal railings. When I say 'metal railings', though, they more closely resembled the crash barriers on the fast lane of a motorway, used to prevent cars crossing onto the wrong side of a carriageway. Although, in our case, it was to keep a hypersexualised boar in *his* own lane and not crossing onto the wrong side of the farm gate.

'Trust me, he'll fly round t'corner where you're stood now,' Kate shouted towards us as she released the beast. 'If yer in his way, he'll tek yer straight off yer feet.'

With Helen and I dressed in our worst clothes underneath navy-blue boiler suits, we stood as spectators behind the safety of the barrier to await the arrival of the rampant boar. The grunting came first. Then the smell. I adore pigs, but I have no shame in accusing them of some pretty intense body odour. The smell of a testosterone-fuelled boar can only be likened to that of the men's urinal on the final day of Glastonbury, an acidic, ammonia smell that permeated the air as he charged along the path in search of his mate.

White saliva frothed from the corners of his mouth. Like bubble bath, it dripped from the yellow tusks that protruded from his mandible as he hurtled towards the sow. His one-track mind was not focused on any courting ritual. There was no poetic Attenborough-esque respectful display of affection. Instead, the boar was in it for one reason, and one reason only. His own primal gratification.

As Helen and I looked on in horror, Kate suddenly appeared jogging along the same racetrack ten feet behind him. 'He's gorrit! He's picked up her scent!' Kate said, slightly out of breath as she jogged along behind the wobbling pair of ginormous testicles. She was clutching a greasy rag in one hand and a large white can that looked like a tin of air freshener in the other, although instead of the words 'Alpine

Fresh', it had in capital letters the words 'BOAR SPRAY' blazoned across the label.

Moments earlier we had used this 'boar spray' to detect which of the sows might have been the most in heat. Helen had spritzed the aerosol directly onto the sow's snout while I had clambered 'side saddle' onto the sow's back to test if she would stand to 'back pressure'. The sow would then either run for the hills (and send me tumbling) or she would stay perfectly still, arch her back a little and allow me to take the weight off my own feet – the latter indicated that she was in peak heat for ovulation, and therefore ready to be mated.

The boar, though, required no such nonsense. He could already sense she was ready. He raced along his 'shag track' and eventually the two animals met. He rose onto his hind legs and climbed up onto the sow's back, his front hooves scratching against the skin of her shoulder blades as he fought to keep his balance.

'Right, put yer glove on,' Kate shouted over to us. 'Who's going first?'

What? Helen and I looked at each other. As two young vet students, neither of us quite knew what was about to happen, or what we had signed up for. We could see in each other's eyes that neither of us particularly wanted to leave the safe sanctuary of the spectators' stand. 'Err, well, I mean ...' I paused, and looked at Helen. 'I s'pose I don't mind, if it's ...' I said, nervously.

'Right you are!' Kate replied. She acknowledged my stuttering as volunteering. 'So, the thing is, he won't be able to find the hole on his own,' she said, peering between the six-foot heap of thrusting pig-on-pig action before us. 'And if he does find it,' she continued, 'it'll probably be t'wrong 'un! So we'll 'av to *guide* him in.'

On the word 'guide', she simultaneously raised her gloved right hand.

I looked at Helen, the two of us stunned into silence, frozen on the spot. I then looked down at the latex glove covering my own right hand. Things were about to get awkward. Weird. And, to my great fear, *intimate*.

Fed up with our polite, passive indecisiveness, Kate decided I was up first. 'Right, c'mon, James . . .'

I felt like the PE teacher had just called my name at school. An adrenaline bolt shot from my stomach. I looked back at Helen. As my teammate, she nodded me into the 'game' with a conviction and pride as if to say, 'C'mon, you've got this!'

'You need to reach down, see if you can grab his penis and then direct it in,' Kate instructed.

Jeez, I thought to myself, contemplating whether it were too late to back out.

The pig's penis, shaped like a corkscrew, was flailing around in the air with a mind of its own as he tried to locate the sow. Where everything is 'placed' anatomically, though, made it seem rather a miracle that any pigs have ever mated successfully in the history of piggy evolution. The physicality of it all just seemed impossible. And further, with each failed attempt at 'target practice', the boar followed through to the finish line regardless, like a child let loose at a summer party with a water pistol. Perhaps one reason why male pigs can produce a colossal half litre of semen: to compensate for the huge quantity of 'waste' that was being fired past me with each thrust of the boar's hips.

I rolled up my sleeve and reached my hand between the

pounding porcine loins, and in doing so I suddenly felt something wet and firm prod against the skin of my forearm. As though trying to grab an eel darting around underwater, I started leaping my hand forwards and backwards trying to grab a hold of the slippery sucker.

I learnt something that day. Firstly, that the life of a pig farmer was perhaps not for me – I am not at all ashamed to say – as I had to relinquish my duties back to Kate before the boar's tank ran dry. And secondly, that I, like many, have a 'concentration face'. I was concentrating so hard on the 'matter in hand' (probably in an attempt to take my mind off what was *actually* in my hand) that I had a facial expression that my mother would say made me look like 'a gormless codfish'. There was one final piece of crucial advice to come from Kate, something I have never forgotten through working with many animals since. Over the din of grunts and squeals, she clocked my expression and shouted, 'Oi! You might wanna keep that gawping mouth o'yours shut, James!' Then laughed along as the boar's flailing corkscrew and his erratic aim continued to pump his piggy love-juice straight past me in every which direction.

It was an important process – to spend time on the various farm placements, in the practical sessions and through the lectures to gain the skills on how to read an animal's body language, how to approach them, better understand their natural behaviour and get to grips with their management (no pun intended). The purpose, though, was to gain a thorough understanding of what 'normal' looked like. Once normal has been appreciated, so the 'abnormal' can be distinguished, then diagnosed and ultimately *hopefully* treated. However, before getting to the 'treatment' part of proceedings, we had to be able to spot the disease itself.

Clinical pathology dominated the fourth year of the degree – this is essentially the study of disease, obtaining samples of tissue and blood to understand how and why an animal has passed away. Or, perhaps a more commonly recognised term is 'post-mortem'. It is a crucial step in veterinary education and requires the 'medical' brain to override the 'emotional' brain to seek clues and answers to the 'whys' and 'hows' of an animal's fatal disease process.

Veterinary medicine has taught me so many lessons – way beyond that of the syllabus or curriculum – and the pathology lab is a place where I had to quickly come to terms with death. Understanding death as a process is a crucial and necessary aspect of understanding veterinary medicine.

The pathology lab was unlike any other room I had ever entered. It commanded a level of respect. It forced a hushed silence on the living students that entered, out of respect for the deceased animals that passed through. A huge white space, like stepping inside a giant plastic box, with speckled blue lino that sloped gently to a grated drain in the middle of the floor. Built like a giant wet room, it allowed for a thorough hose-down in between each investigative procedure to wash away the detritus and disease from one deceased animal before the next one arrived. It felt like being at a dockyard – a chain and winch system hung suspended from the ceiling across a framework of steel girders flanked by two huge doors, tall enough to allow a lorry to reverse up to them and the vast, cavernous chamber created a sound all of its own – a loud acoustic echo, the clanging of chains, the clunking mechanical action of the winch, the booming slam of the double doors and the voice of a clinician talking about matters of veterinary pathology. It should have been a fascinating insight into the study of disease, but I could never quite feel able to concentrate. It wasn't a pleasant space to be in. And I came to dread every single session.

My first experience of the pathology lab was the post-mortem exam of a large racehorse – winched through the doors on the huge crane from the back of a truck and gently laid out before us on the industrial stainless-steel table. Clad in white lab coats and wellington boots, the twenty or so students crowded round with clipboards and an eagerness to uncover the true cause of death – like an animal version of *Silent Witness*. The horse's abdomen was swollen, really swollen – almost as though someone had taken a giant balloon pump and inflated it to the point of lift off. But the swelling wasn't air – as the lecturer was about to reveal, with one clean swipe of the blade in her hand. Instead of air, a huge torrent of yellow, creamy, custard pus flowed like a slow, serene waterfall from the abdomen. It filled the tabletop, breached the boundaries, flooded the floor, then meandered its way down the gentle gradient towards the drain before it glooped through the metal grate. Pus. Some vets love the stuff – the satisfying 'pop' of a cat bite abscess, the draining fountain from the back of a cow's leg, the rotten tooth root of a dog. All extremely satisfying to diagnose and treat, there is no denying. But one thing that you can never quite prepare for is how you'll react to the gut-wrenching smell. I learnt that for me, it was not at all well.

This was the point at which the horse had to be turned over. The mechanics of the crane clunked back into action and the dripping carcass began to elevate until it hung suspended in mid-air. As the winch turned, the momentum caused it to swing slowly, and it crept closer and closer towards me. Then the putrid, fetid smell hit me and I could stomach no more. The combination of the smell, the death, the pus and the white lab coats suddenly triggered a wave of nausea I have never known before. I had no choice but to run, as fast I could, to the gents' toilets and vomit.

I failed clinical pathology, perhaps unsurprisingly.

But while I was instructed to keep my mouth shut on a pig farm, in the pathology lab the opposite applied. The revolutionary tip from the pathology lecturer to try breathing through an open mouth – 'it doesn't smell so bad if you don't use your nose!' – got me back through the door and into the room. I also applied Olbas Oil to the inside of my nostrils (the sting was worth it to drown the stench), in an attempt to recondition my brain into believing all dead animals smell of menthol and eucalyptus. The only way forwards was to find a way to cope. And with these little tips under my belt, I passed the resit. Although I still don't cope well with pus.

However, eventually came the fifth and final year. A chance to amalgamate all the learnt knowledge and begin our clinical rotations. Assisting in the treatment of the real, living and breathing animals we were helping to save, under the watchful tuition of the professors. The final year still mainly revolved around a lot of shadowing the senior clinicians but it also allowed some increased clinical freedoms, the chance to get a little more involved – like a group of toddlers let loose in the playground, but still with reins on for anyone thinking they could run before they could walk.

On the surgical rotation, we stood and observed groundbreaking procedures. After half an hour of scrubbing our palms and between our fingers with the plastic bristles of a firm scrubbing brush, we then splashed our bright red hands with an eye-wateringly volatile antiseptic solution before pushing them into sterile latex gloves, all while dressed head to toe in sterile gowns, hats and masks. Each of us sweated buckets as we stood like lemons around the surgeon and watched as she operated on a paralysed dachshund's spine, a procedure known as a hemilaminectomy, to relieve the pressure from the ruptured intervertebral disc that had buckled under the strain of the sausage dog's elongated back. A huge pale blue surgical drape covered the entire body of the little sausage dog, trailed beyond the edges of the operating table and almost to the floor. Like an enormous bedsheet with a tiny window no bigger than a postage stamp cut into it, through which the operation was performed. None of us could see a thing. However, to test our attention span, occasionally one of us would be called upon individually to pass an instrument. The pressure on that student not to drop the metal, specialist and, crucially, sterile piece of equipment was immense as the instrument was lifted from the surgeon's tray, carried through the air and placed into the open palm of the surgeon's gloved hand. It felt like greeting royalty, to gift directly into the hands of the powers that be, then bow your head and take one firm step back. The biggest fear, though, was the gamble on whether you'd actually picked up the correct bit of kit – learning the names of the hundreds of individual items of surgical instrumentation almost required a degree in its own right. Imagine the fear – 'pass me the Caspar modular self-retaining retractor, please' – as my hand hovered tentatively over the plethora of instruments.

Dermatology was all about the products: supplements, skin creams and shampoos. It was a bit like working in the health and beauty section of a department store, but for pets. It also involved a lot of time spent looking down the microscope, which made me feel like I had motion sickness. Hours spent staring down the lens in search of bugs that had been plucked, scraped or swabbed from the groin, feet or ears of whichever scabby, itchy or balding creature had visited the skin clinic that morning. The aim was to differentiate between a parasitic, fungal or bacterial cause of the skin complaint. Like a veterinary version of Cluedo – which bug is it? Where on the animal's body was it found? And what weapon could we use to kill it? However, confusion erupted one session on finding a smattering of unusual yet unmistakable tadpole-shaped cells on a swab collected from an infected ear. At the gawps and yells from the eager students who discovered it, everyone collected around the microscope to see for themselves. Fingers started to point, tongues began to wag. Conclusions drawn through many an elaborate hypothesis. True enough, a sperm cell among dots of bacteria, all dug out together from the depths of a cat's ear canal.

Only later, after the rumours had already flooded our campus social networking site, did we find out that the student rotation group that had used the teaching room before ours was the canine reproduction group, who had quite spectacularly failed to replenish the pots of 'diff quick' stain (a solution used to transform the translucent cells on a slide into visible blue or pink shapes when viewed under a microscope). As their slides got dipped into each pot of stain, a few cells got left behind, so that when our subsequent dermatology slides were dipped into the same pots a few hours later, they were essentially being plunged into a soup of doggy sperm cells. I often think about that poor cat owner, a very lovely man who is still blissfully unaware that at one point he had an entire year group of wildly over-imaginative vet students speculating over whether whatever he practised behind closed doors may, or may not, have contributed to his cat's ear infection!

After dermatology, we had three weeks on ICU – twenty-one days of twenty-four-hour shifts monitoring and medicating the sickest pets. Those recovering from the aforementioned spinal surgery, for example; animals who would remain in a state of paralysis post-operatively for many days and would need to be turned every few hours. Cats who had lengths of intestines surgically removed, or those that screamed in pain from a blood clot lodged in their inner thigh, or couldn't go to the toilet due to a smashed pelvis after a run-in with a car tyre. Dogs with infectious diseases that required isolation, livers that had twisted, stomachs that had bloated, spleens that had ruptured, fevers that couldn't be explained. Or animals that had arrived collapsed or wouldn't stop fitting. The sickest patients came through the intensive care unit and the admissions could happen anytime, twenty-four hours a day. The radio played dance hits, the kettle remained boiled and caffeine was consumed in vast quantities.

The small animal practice rotation had a much slower pace and offered students the chance to play at being a real GP vet with real clients and real animals. This was where we learnt about the routine healthcare of pets – like vaccinations or vomiting bugs, over- or under-active thyroid glands, or how to deal with sloppy stools. Any pet with a minor ailment could be treated in the small animal practice. Here we were allowed to get a little more hands on – taking blood samples, administering vaccinations or checking pet's teeth. While not a perk of the job, an essential skill usually mastered early on in one's veterinary career is to get to grips with how to express a dog's anal glands (two scent glands found just inside a dog's bottom). Some dogs require this procedure on a fairly regular basis – it often becomes quite an obsession of many owners, somewhat understandably, as the smell of leaking glands around the house is particularly repugnant. Especially if the dog is the size of a small horse, with a penchant for sitting on his owner's lap.

A regular visitor to the small animal practice was a Great Dane called Hank, who could somehow fold himself up to sit neatly on the cream leather passenger seat of his owner's convertible Jaguar. We could spot them coming a mile off, and it often looked as though Hank himself was behind the steering wheel, driving himself to the vet's for a quick 'bum squeeze'. As Hank pulled into the car park on this particular visit, it was my turn to meet him and offer a helping hand with his blocked-up back end. The glove went on, the enormous gland was felt and despite his owner pleading (somewhat proudly) that her dog's glands were 'usually very difficult for most students to express', with one determined squish between finger and thumb, an explosion of fishy, dark brown glandular material came spraying out. It ejected with such an almighty force that it fired straight past my gloved hand and the clump of cotton wool clutched in my palm, up my arm, across my glasses and through my hair – and then splattered a huge brown 'rainbow' arch along the painted white wall of the consulting room, reaching almost to the height of the wooden door frame. I wiped the lens of my glasses and looked at the owner, whose facial expression was stuck somewhere between impressed and horrified before she uttered, 'Good grief! Well . . . you're clearly a *very* good squirter!' Hank looked a little less impressed. I thanked her, and as they left the room, I sat on the consult-room chair trying to work out my next conundrum: how to rinse the sprayed-on gland juice from my hair and uniform without plunging my entire head under the running tap. I tried my best in the circumstances, but I think it's fair to say the distinct aroma surreptitiously lurked around me for the rest of that day.

Gaining 'hands on' experience is one thing, but as vets we often go for a 'hands in' approach too, if possible. Never truer than when it comes to the pregnancy diagnosis of a herd of dairy cows on our farm rotation. A row of twenty eager vet students, standing behind a row of dairy cows, an arm-length plastic glove on one hand and a bottle of lube the size of a milk bottle being passed down the line in the other. On the count of three, each tail was lifted and a well-lubed gloved hand inserted. It is the question every vet student gets asked – 'have you had to put your hand up a cow's bum?' Absolutely. Sometimes the only way is to have a good feel inside. Cow, sheep, horse, dog, even the occasional chicken needs her cloaca checking from time to time, and who better suited than the gloved index finger of a willing veterinarian? It is a rite of passage that we get to know our patients inside and out. Every vet student is taught this important procedure to feel for a pregnancy, gently assessing the size and shape of the cow's ovaries. Or to pass the probe of an ultrasound scanning machine in to have a good look around, the grey and white grainy image displayed on the screen of a small box about the size of a bread bin encased in a royal-blue plastic case to protect the expensive machinery from any sudden falling cowpats. Standing outside for hours on a freezing cold Wednesday afternoon, with my fingers numb and frozen, I've never been more grateful than the moment my cow passed a huge waterfall of sloppy dung – *warm* sloppy dung. It was then I realised I could plunge my gloved hand into the freshly laid, steaming hot cowpat to defrost my hands and bring some sensation back to my fingertips. Like a farmyard version of one of those teabag-style hand warmers hikers take up a mountain – just a bit wetter. I'll confess to you now, those arm-length gloves are made of very thin plastic. But it was a case of needs must. And I'd put money on it that you'd do the same if you were in my wellies!

The veterinary syllabus was a true baptism of fire. I could never have predicted the onslaught of knowledge this in-depth education would give me. From a tortoise to a Shire horse, and every creature in between, we had to discover and understand all about the inner workings of every animal. I could also never have imagined the copious amounts of bodily fluids I would get comfortable with – and covered with – or learn to deal with the smell of. It was an education in so many different ways. I tried to absorb every morsel of clinical information we were given over that gruelling five-year course. But as I look back now, I see that everything I learnt through vet school was really just the beginning. There were many more lessons yet to come.

CHAPTER 3

Samuel

June, 2007

The mobile phone on the passenger seat next to me suddenly sprang into life – vibrating, flashing, screaming to tell me it was precisely 1.15 p.m. An image of my fellow vet school friends with their bright, drunken smiles shone from the home screen, reminding me of happier times. I pressed and held the power button until eventually the phone surrendered. Our drunk smiles faded as the alarm fell silent and the screen turned to black. *It's time*, I told myself. A bolt of nervous energy radiated from my stomach.

With only five minutes to spare, I stepped out from the safe haven of my clapped-out Vauxhall Corsa. A familiar scent of disinfectant wafted from the soles of my wellington boots as I pulled them from their plastic carrier bag. A meticulous scrubbing session the evening before (involving a bucket of diluted iodine and an old toothbrush) made sure every garment gleamed – from the boots on my feet to the swamp-green overalls folded neatly on the back seat. I placed my wellington boots on the floor and loosened my trainers.

Supporting myself on the car door frame, I lifted each leg in turn and pulled on the over-trousers before plunging each foot down into the heel of a wellington boot. I then pushed my head up and through the high-necked smock, before working my clenched fists through the elasticated armbands of each short sleeve, creating a torniquet around each bicep so tight that I could feel my fingers swell with the nerves and pressure.

It was not only my clinical knowledge that was about to undergo scrutiny; as the classified email had highlighted, my physical appearance was equally important:

> *Veterinary students should arrive at the farm at their allocated time. Please do not arrive early as there may still be an examination in progress. For biosecurity reasons, please wear appropriate, clean protective clothing and waterproof boots that can be disinfected on arrival.*

The purpose of this impermeable veterinary outerwear was to allow one's gloved arm to enter the backside of an animal, a messy affair at best, which usually required a full-body hose-down afterwards.

My adrenaline-soaked heart pounded like a drum as I stood dressed head to toe in my green overalls. The School of Veterinary Sciences was our base for the last two out of five years of our university teaching. At the centre of the campus stood a tired yet charming Victorian mansion, repurposed from her early days as a magnificent country home. This now served as the iconic central 'veterinary headquarters'.

I left my car and started my walk across the campus towards the university farm. The wide former driveway gently snaked away from the mansion, through the (previously) formal gardens and out onto a sleepy country lane. The original driveway entrance, no longer in use, was adorned by two large rusting iron gates held slightly ajar by a padlocked chain. There was just enough slack to allow a vet student to sneak between and clamber through a few years of overgrowth and weeds. Usually a shortcut to the pub, it *also* deposited the adventurous, trail-finding vet student directly at the university farm entrance.

As I walked, the warm smell of summer filled the air. It was an unusually hot day in June. There was nothing I craved more than to lie my weary body (and mind) down in the tall swaying grass and relax in the sun. After the pressure of our final year of clinical rotations, I could no longer remember how to simply stop, or relax. I had spent months at my desk trawling through countless past exam papers stacked high among the animal-themed textbooks. I lived off caffeine and bags of Fruit Pastilles, sent through the mail with a postcard from my mother that invariably had the words 'keep your pecker up' scribed somewhere in the text.

Time was irrelevant. The days were not divided by hours but instead by subject matter on a scribbled revision timetable. Fresh air had become a distant memory. My room hummed with a musky scent of student neglect. The sheets on my unmade bed had relinquished their crisp ivory glory to a tone I can only describe as 'sebaceous beige'. Discarded Pot Noodle containers. Abandoned mugs of tea. Unwashed dinner plates. All sat like petri dishes in a laboratory, culturing a disc of furry mould across their surface like a microbiologist's

41

playground. This was not a healthy existence. But it was my way of 'revising'.

Each student sat five final spoken exams in total, over the course of two or three weeks, focusing on the broad pillars of veterinary medicine – canine, feline, farm, equine and veterinary public health. Five long years of study coming to an end. I had reached the final furlong, exhausted. And now I needed to find some Goliath strength to complete this last exam and hopefully accomplish my lifelong dream to become a vet.

As I reached the end of the driveway, I slid sideways through the narrow gap created between the two arms of the open iron gates and, in doing so, brushed against the large moss-covered iron latch. I felt the latch scrape along my chest. It smeared an earthy, rusty stain across my pristine overall. I tried to wipe it away with my nervous palm, but it only smudged further. *Shit! No, no, no!* the only words darting around in my head as I continued to wipe. Less than a minute until exam time. Five long years of veterinary education boycotted by the skid mark of a rusting iron gate across my front.

A large-framed man, wearing a chequered shirt and a maroon tie, beckoned me over. He had broad shoulders down to a full waist, with sleeves rolled to the elbows, stone-coloured chinos and a pair of forest-green wellington boots. He was a senior clinician of the Vet School Farm Department, well respected but with a notoriously intimidating examination style. His maroon tie showcased the silhouette of a cow, embroidered in gold thread, sitting perfectly at the level of his heart. Exemplary farm vet attire.

'Greenwood?' After weeks of solitude and silence, his voice boomed in my ears.

'Yes,' I replied, in a broken, awkward squawk, and simultaneously raised my hand in the air like a kindergarten child.

The afternoon sun had now reached its peak. Beads of nervous sweat bubbled on my forehead as I sweltered in my PVC overalls. He surveyed my appearance. I began by hastily apologising and justifying the offensive smear across my torso. 'It has literally just happened.' I pointed to the gate, with an apologetic plea.

I awaited his verdict. Then he ticked a box on the piece of paper attached to the clipboard he was holding and said, 'OK, follow me.'

I was in.

We turned and walked towards the barn, but I had no idea of what was to come. *Cows*, I said to myself, as I followed two or three steps behind, trying to arrange my thoughts and maintain composure, *it must be cows*. The long, deep bellows of a herd of dairy cows echoed from the cool, dark barn ahead of us. Conversing among themselves, as though placing bets on each student.

I attempted to mentally visualise the pages of my cattle notes. Diagrams, flow charts, acronyms all jumbled themselves into formulas and sentences that made absolutely no sense. Panic had absolutely taken hold. The oral exams were particularly ruthless. Any question, about any animal, asked there and then on the spot. It felt as though my fledgling veterinary knowledge was about to be hauled up on the butcher's block, as well as my own future.

We both entered the large barn and my eyes adjusted to the near darkness. In the shadows, flanked by two rows of cattle stalls, a second man was standing beside a wooden trestle table adorned with various pieces of farm equipment.

Birthing ropes, silver packets of powdered electrolytes, various bottles of drugs, needles, syringes, stomach tubes and a pile of photographs showing a variety of ailing livestock. The second man was a practising farm vet drafted in from a highly successful practice in Shropshire. He briefly curled one side of his upper lip into a half-smile as I was introduced, then quickly dropped it in a 'let's get straight down to business' kind of way.

I was instructed to take a moment and consider the table in front of me. 'The examination begins now; the time is one twenty-one p.m.'

As he said it, the row of cows behind me shuffled their feet to gather around and take a closer look. One or two belted out the occasional 'moooo' as they all strained their necks over the metal chain across the central walkway of the barn. They sniffed the air around me and occasionally revealed a huge grey prehensile tongue as they tried to reach and lick my arm. That is, until I moved, and the herd would jolt back a few feet before slowly creeping forwards again.

My interrogation began with an imaginary scenario: a pig farmer had turned up at the practice I was working at, asking for some antibiotics for his coughing sows. Surrounded by cows but being asked about pigs. Not cows. I was thrown into immediate confusion from the start.

'Right,' I replied, stunned into silence, frantically scrolling through to the pig lecture notes in my mind.

He held out both of his hands and hovered them over the table as he spoke. 'This is what you have available in the pharmacy.'

A collection of glass bottles contained injectable liquid medicines of various colours – bright sunshine yellow, opaque white, magenta, clear – all arranged in neat rows, out of the direct sunlight in this fictitious animal apothecary.

'And finally, James, my question is, what are you going to do?'

Over to me. I started inspecting the various bottles. Small strips of black duct tape had been used to cover any dosing guidelines or indications for use, leaving only the active ingredient but no trade name visible.*

'Well. I would like to check that these pigs are under our care. Have we been to this farm before?' I cautiously replied.†

Was I genuinely attempting to shut down his line of questioning on a technicality? A risky strategy. But it might buy me some time.

'Yes, they are indeed under your care.'

I smiled.

I dropped my gaze back to the table and spotted an opportunity. A glass bottle with a ruby-red metallic collar

---

* Every licensed medicine has two names – the trade name and the active ingredient. For example, in human medicine, 'Nurofen' would be an example of a trade name for the active ingredient ibuprofen. Most vets in practice will refer to drugs by their trade name in day-to-day conversations. A vet student picks up most of their knowledge on drug selection through seeing practice, while the teaching universities only ever refer to drugs by the active ingredient. However, a medicine with the same active ingredient could be sold under four or five (or more) different trade names. And each drug will only be licensed for a specific number of animal species and diseases. Trying to memorise all these variations is a huge challenge for most undergraduate vet students, especially under examination conditions.

† Veterinarians are only permitted to prescribe medications to animals that are registered as being 'under their care'.

showcased a translucent, golden elixir. As I carefully gripped on to the metal collar of the bottle neck, I felt a surge of confidence. I held up the offering. 'Tylosin,' I said. 'This is the only antibiotic on the table licensed for pigs and is indicated for the treatment of swine pneumonia,' I explained, with an eloquent efficiency. Surely this was the answer he was searching for?

He pulled his lips wide, leant forwards and took the bottle from me and rotated it in his hands. I watched the last few millilitres swishing around inside the vial. He held up the bottle with only a centimetre or so of liquid left. 'Not even enough to treat a single pig in there. What else?'

A spontaneous twist in his porcine narrative. He held the confiscated bottle behind his back and nodded me back into the game. Nothing was registering. The other antibiotics were only licensed for use in sheep or cows. Perhaps this was his tactic, to lead me into a discussion around the use of drugs across different species, the legislation, the cascade rules, the various withdrawal times if those animals might eventually enter the human food chain. Perhaps he wanted me to ask the fictitious farmer some more questions? Perhaps I should offer to see the pigs. YES. I should insist that I needed to examine the sows in person.

I stood firm in my defence. Safeguarding against the flippant dispensing of antibiotics was 'modern thinking' back then and might have earned me some brownie points. It didn't. And it was not the answer he was fishing for.

'So he's driven all the way to the practice and you're not going to offer him *anything*?'

'Not until I've examined at least one pig.' I stood my ground.

'Right. Well. In that case . . .'

He kept the clipboard tilted towards his torso and out of my vision. He wrinkled his face up into an 'oh deary me' look while his hand followed a piece of string to a biro pen. He took the pen and struck a long line across the entire page, corner to corner, followed by the sharp stab of a full stop. A whole section of the exam had just been discarded.

My mouth dried. Meanwhile, elsewhere, the sweat cascaded. My armpits, back and neck were drenched. I immediately regretted my wardrobe choice. I too was sporting a shirt, tie and thick corduroy trousers hidden underneath the impermeable plastic outerwear. And right then I wished I had followed the tactics of my braver housemate, who attended his exam in only his boxer shorts under his overalls, knowing full well no one would *actually* check.

The tension was unbearable.

Picture flashcards came next – photographs of various cows suffering with various ailments, held up individually like the 'A is for Apple' training cards parents use with toddlers, except the 'A', in this case, was for a cow's 'abomasal volvulus'. The row of *actual* cows behind me continued to strain their inquisitive gaze over my shoulder to see whatever was going on, almost as though they were trying to look at the picture flashcards themselves. It wouldn't have surprised me if they'd recognised a friend or two. 'Oooh, eh, look, that one's of you, Daisy!'

It was then time to move on. I left behind the gaggle of supportive nosy cows and followed the two men through the large open doors of the cow barn. We emerged like reptiles into the warming ultraviolet sunlight and crossed to the opposite side of the walled farmyard where a set of galvanised hurdles had been arranged into a makeshift pen. A large sheet of royal-blue tarpaulin was stretched over some piled hay bales to create some shade for whatever creature lurked within. A plastic laminated sheet of A4 paper had the name 'Samuel' typed in thick black ink, and had been attached to the metal hurdle with a couple of cable ties.

As we approached, I could just make out a mound of creamy woolly fleece that poked out from behind one of the hay bales. We'd been spotted. A well-muscled ram jumped to his feet and left the shaded sanctuary of his hay bales behind. He darted as fast as he could to the furthest corner of the pen, then stood perfectly square and stared right at the three of us. Our disruption to his afternoon nap triggered his own sudden bolt of nervous energy as he widened his hind limbs, stamped his front foot and released a torrent of pee.

'Can you tell me what breed Samuel here is?' enquired the second examiner, his turn now, as he nodded his head towards the ram. A slim man, tall, with an open-necked chequered shirt and the obligatory stone-coloured chinos. He was younger and spoke much quieter, with a very slight hint of a Welsh accent. He almost seemed nervous himself to be paired up with the veterinary heavyweight standing next to him. Perhaps he was an ex-student? Perhaps this was his first stint as an examiner? Either way, it felt as though he was also out to prove himself.

'He's a Texel,' I replied. *Hard to forget the look of a Texel.*

'Good. Hop in and catch him up.' He handed me a rope with a series of loops and knots.

I climbed over one of the metal hurdles and into the octagonal pen. The two men looked on from the sidelines of this makeshift arena, acting like Julius Caesar and his li'l buddy. My job was to wrestle the beast, entertain, prove my worth – and for them, they got to judge whatever spectacle was about to unfold before them. With arms outstretched, head down and knees slightly bent, I edged towards the ram, creeping step by step like a confident seagull approaching a discarded bag of chips at the seaside.

I quietly muttered the words 'good lad' over and over (perhaps calming myself down more than the ram). As I stepped closer, his ears started to twitch. A nervous tension escalated between us. He swung his head to the left and then right. He was plotting, looking for an escape route around me. He was young, ballsy and his instinct was telling him to run. I had naively hoped he might've been open to a negotiation, that with a shake of hand and hoof, he might step into the head halter so we could then take a bow to the standing ovation from our onlookers. Sadly, I was wrong.

With only about a metre left between us, it was time for me to commit. I lunged forwards and stepped my left knee in front of his shoulder, plunged my fingertips deep into his thick, oily fleece and clung on for dear life. Instead of my left leg acting like a barrier, though, it hinged and swung open like the starting gate on a horse racetrack and he ran straight past.

With lightning speed, the ram started to do laps of the pen. Unwilling to let go, he dragged me along with him. He darted round and round the pen like an out-of-control speedboat with me lolloping, skipping, stumbling and flying along with him. On the third lap of the pen I managed to get one step ahead of him and with an almighty heave I backed him into a corner, pushed my knee in front of his shoulder and pulled one of the hurdles close to his side. I just about managed to wrap the halter over his nose and round the back of his head and we both stood still. Fighting to catch my breath, I held tightly on to the long end of rope. As soon as the head halter was on, the ram's mood shifted completely as though his brief performance of non-compliance was just an elaborate part of a staged theatrical plan all along.

But what now?

'Got there eventually,' I heard coming from the other side of the metal hurdles.

'Right then, talk me through how you would perform a clinical exam of this ram.'

I took a deep breath. 'I'd start with the nose. I'm looking for any discharge,' I said, kneeling face to face with the ram, his chin in one hand and me pointing at each nostril in turn with the other.

I then stroked my hand along his bony mandible. 'I'm now feeling along the jawline and—'

'Why are you feeling along the jawline?' the vet interjected.

'Well, for example, if there are any swellings, or—'

'And why might there be a swelling?' he interjected, *again*.

'Err, there might be an abscess in the tooth root, a cancer or maybe an infection in one of his lymph nodes which are—'

'How might a sheep get an infection in a lymph node?' he pinged back.

I tried to remain calm. Focused. There was no denying, though, that being interrupted at every turn was infuriatingly off-putting. *They just want to get the most information out of you*, said my older sister's voice in my head, a calming reminder to stay cool and just 'play the game'.

Luckily, though, 'caseous lymphadenitis' in sheep was the most recent topic on my revision plan. In my quick-minded manipulation of the situation, I had intentionally dropped some 'lymph node' bait and the examining vet had gobbled it up. The player had just got played. I explained the condition in detail while using up as much time as I could. A highly contagious bacterial infection among sheep and goats that will inevitably form an abscess in the lymph node. The likelihood being, specifically with rams, that he probably contracted the infection through headbutting other rams, leaving them both with bloody battle scars. The men both looked cautiously impressed.

We moved on. Eyes, ears, spine, neck, and then to the chest. 'I would check the respiratory rate and the rhythm of breathing.'

I talked through what would be normal for a sheep's lung and what would be classed as abnormal – crackles, wheezes and popping sounds. I mumbled an explanation of what 'adventitious' meant and took the focus onto coughing. And that a cough could be due to a build-up of fluid in or around the lungs.

'And what could the fluid be around the lungs?' he interrupted, back to his usual tricks.

'Err, it could be anything from blood to pus, maybe chyle . . .'

Of course, his next question: 'And what is chyle?'

Bollocks. I had just thrown myself under a very large tractor-shaped bus.

OK, so here's the thing. Chyle is a difficult topic to explain. And chyle in the chest is even more difficult to explain.

Essentially, a chylothorax is where lymph (the component of blood that gets left behind when the blood seeps into the tissues to nourish them) has formed in the digestive tract (now chyle) and then accumulates in the chest (aka thorax). All important, but also not particularly thrilling to get one's head around. Especially when there are plenty more exciting things to learn about like caesarean sections or how to contain a potentially catastrophic disease outbreak or how to rescue a horse from a ditch with the fire brigade. So, in my head, lymph and chyle got clumped together and thrown on the boring miscellaneous pile as just 'stuff'. As in 'stuff' that probably won't come up in an exam. Now, though, that reckless abandonment had come back to haunt me. And, at that moment, the most inexplicable sentence somehow escaped my frazzled brain, travelled down various frazzled synaptic pathways and spewed from my then very frazzled mouth: 'Chyle . . . is . . . the ectopic . . . lymphatic . . . cytoplasm . . . of . . . plasma.'

Woah, what . . . what was THAT? I thought to myself. With one hand gripping on to the head halter, the other pressed against the sheep's chest, I looked up from the urine-soaked straw I was kneeling in.

The examiner just stared blankly before he took a deep breath in to speak . . . but before he could: 'WAIT!' I exclaimed, loudly. We all jumped, even the ram.

'That bit doesn't count!' I insisted.

WHAT WAS HAPPENING? Why were these words cascading from my mouth?

The examiner paused in disbelief. His facial expression turned from shock to exasperation.

'James,' he paused, 'firstly, let me remind you that this is an examination.' I nodded apologetically. 'And secondly, that last sentence can't count as it . . . does . . . not . . . make . . . any . . . logical . . . sense!' the vet replied.

I hung my head, accepting defeat and, right at that moment, a buzzer sounded signalling that my time was up. The end. No further chances. Nothing more that could be said or done and I was asked to leave the farm.

I thanked both the men with a handshake, crossed the heat of the yard and walked back towards the lane. At the farm gate I turned back, only briefly, to see if I could glimpse their reaction. The ram had reclaimed his afternoon shade and the two men were walking side by side, back towards the cool sanctuary of the cattle shed, both laughing together and shaking their heads. My heart sank.

I kicked the stone wall of the farmyard entrance, annoyed at myself that I'd let my nerves get the better of me. I'd completely messed it up. As I walked up the lane, I pulled the overall back up and over my head, untucked my soaked shirt and pinched the thin layer of sodden cotton fabric from the small of my back before loosening the tie around my neck. A light breeze cooled my skin as I slowly meandered back to my car.

Now, as the adrenaline in my heart dissolved away and the anxious fog that clogged my mind slowly cleared, all my stored clinical knowledge came flooding back. I replayed each question in my mind, over and over, thinking how differently I should have answered. And how much detail I had left out. But more frustratingly, I realised how much I had answered incorrectly.

It would be six long weeks before the exam results would be published, and as I drove off it hit me that there was nothing more I could do than wait. It was only a short drive back to our student digs. Out of the four other guys I lived with, I was the last to finish exams. As I stepped through the door, an almighty roar blasted from the living room. The rugby union summer internationals were in full swing and the four of them were fully engrossed, topless, cheering at the television screen and analysing the game. Empty cans of beer lay strewn across the carpet and a large bucket of ice kept the unopened ones cool (it was at least thirty degrees outside). After months of silence and frayed tempers under the stress of exams – normal student life had suddenly resumed.

I crossed the living room and took a seat in the broken charity shop armchair. Andy leant in next to me. Two decades since the day we met, he is still one of my closest friends. 'Hoi did't go?' he asked, with his strong Northern Irish accent.

I shook my head and stared into nothingness. 'Ballsed it up, mate.'

I exhaled with a long, slow and remorseful sigh. I sank into the chintz armchair, placed my elbow on the stained armrest and rested my forehead into my palm. Feeling completely deflated, and wracked with a dreadful disappointment in myself, a lump swelled in my throat as I fought hard to hold back the tears.

Andy stood up. He walked to the ice bucket in the middle of the room and pulled out two cans of cheap lager. He shook the water from them and then returned.

'Aye, but it's don now! Here.' He handed me one of the cans. We each cracked open the ringpull, waited for the fizz to escape, tapped our cans together and took a long overdue swig of well-deserved ice-cold lager.

As the weeks slowly ticked by, I had received a text message from a friend to say that our final exam results had been published. Of course, a publicly produced list of exam results means everyone can see your results before you've even had a chance to check them for yourself. The gossip was rife.

As I walked along the university corridor of the small animal surgery department, a group of fellow vet students had gathered, huddled around the green felt-covered pin board on the wall where three pieces of white A4 paper had been pinned neatly in the middle. As each student walked up to the board, their grade could almost be predicted just by the look on everyone *else's* face. Eyes glistened with tears of relief as the realisation struck for those that had passed. For others, their story came to an abrupt standstill as tears fell from exhausted red, bloodshot eyes for those that had not achieved the required pass mark. The entire process was pretty traumatic for all, and perhaps explains why, even fifteen years later, I will still occasionally wake from the re-curring 'final exams' nightmare.

I reached the board and began to search. Approximately two thirds of the way down on the first sheet of paper I reached the coded combination of numbers that correlated to my exam paper.

Intial: 'JG'

Code: '4342'

I ran my shaking index finger along the text, as each spoken examination was listed by subject matter. In order to pass, we had to achieve the minimum 50 per cent pass mark across all exams.

Companion Animal: 56%

Equine: 59%

Farm Animal: 50%. *Shit. SHIT.*

My heart rate quickened. I could feel each beat reverber-ate around my chest like a kickdrum, beating into my throat as the blood pumped through my jugular veins, my mouth dried like parched sponge. A close shave, but I was still in with a chance.

Veterinary Public Health: 66%. MERIT. *A merit? Bloody hell!*

Overall grade: Pass.

BLOODY HELL!

I read it again. And again. Pass.

I couldn't believe it. I'd passed. Only just perhaps, but I'd done it. I had passed my final exams – the final step towards realising my ultimate dream in life, to become a vet.

I looked across at a friend. We gave each other a quiet nod then quickly returned outside to celebrate. Our student welfare officer congratulated me. I confessed how convinced I was that I'd failed. He agreed, which was perhaps a little worrying! And said the clinician who had moderated my companion animal viva had never before seen a student as nervous as I was. I laughed. Because it was true. But through the laughter, it also proved just how much this all meant to me. How much I wanted it. How much I cared.

And so, I graduated later that month – a ceremony in which I signed an oath to 'promise and solemnly declare . . . my constant endeavour . . . to ensure the health and welfare of animals committed to my care'. The president of the Royal College of Veterinary Surgeons handed me a degree certificate. I shook his hand. *Finally* I had been granted the ticket to my dream life. I had a veterinary degree in my back pocket and I could take it wherever I wanted.

My overriding memory from vet school was just how much hard work it took to successfully complete each of the five years of study. To become a vet, someone has to really, *really* want to become a vet. No one accidentally falls into veterinary medicine and no one goes into it lightly – it took blood, sweat and tears for me to reach my goal. If you ever hear someone say 'vets are only in it for the money', believe me, as someone who has been through it and seen it all, the very last thing on my mind then and now, as motivation for me to endure five years of *all* that – and to devote my life to caring for animals – was money!

CHAPTER 4

Beth

I looked down at the caramel-coloured Jersey cow lying on her front. Her legs were tucked neatly underneath her, steam bellowed from her nostrils with each heavy pant and the smell of sweet fermentation emitted from her insides. A white mist rose from her sweating body and filled the cold winter's air around her like a bovine aromatherapy diffuser. The barn was pitch black except for Mrs Pallot's offer to switch on the single filament bulb swinging from the wooden rafters overhead. After a few flickers, the faint yellowish glow of the bulb had illuminated the dark space above the cow but little else of the old rickety barn we were both standing in.

Mrs Pallot must have been at least eighty and was dressed in wellington boots, a long raincoat and a wide-rimmed waxed hat. She leant dependently on a sturdy carved wooden shepherd's crook but she could still traverse the uneven terrain of the farmyard as nimbly as the equally aged ginger tom cat that followed in her footsteps. The farm appeared as ancient as she was, yet somehow everything ticked along

– as it always had done – just so. Until Thursday evening came round, at six o'clock, when one of her prized dairy cows decided to fall sick.

On reaching the farm, and checking her over, things didn't quite add up. I pulled out my mobile phone. 'Oh, yeah, h-hi Greg, it's, err, it's just Ja-James . . . I'm with the cow now . . . err, I just won-wondered if I can I just ask you a really quick question?' I asked in a pathetically apologetic tone. I correct new graduates now when I hear them belittle themselves as 'just' before giving their name. 'You are not *just* anyone!' Despite that, though, I can *still* remember how utterly petrifying it is as a new graduate vet to have to phone your boss for help. I had only been in the job for a couple of months, straight out of university and, coupled with that, had an inexplicable phobia of talking on the telephone. Being able to talk on the telephone was one of my biggest hurdles when I first graduated. I would hide away in a quiet office so no one could hear me. Or use the work mobile and sit in my car to report blood results. I still hate it now. So the very idea of having to telephone my boss and ask for a moment of his time felt roughly daunting.

The textbooks taught me that milk fever should be associated with the days around calving, not months later. And my lecture notes taught me to look for the very distinct 'looks like head bent back on chest as though cow looking at own arse' position, which was my scribbled annotation of how to spot hypocalcaemia in a cow, written in black biro at the top right-hand corner of the A4 page of lecture notes. I had the reference texts piled up on the back seat of my car, ready for me to refer to in situations like this, but with the cow's more unusual presentation, they offered little help. I wasn't yet fully versed in the subtle variations from the 'textbook' presentation of the various veterinary ailments.

'I've managed to check her over,' I said sheepishly to Greg. 'I'm pretty sure it's milk fever. She's lying, panting, head's back . . .'

Greg acknowledged my list of symptoms with an 'uh-huh, yeah, sounds 'bout right'.

'Tell him she's been down less than an hour,' Mrs Pallot whispered over me while I spoke. She sounded defensive. Apparently she'd been told not to 'leave things so late' by her son.

'She's been down less than an hour.' I smiled over to her. 'But she calved back in July, which is now about three months ago. I thought milk fever was much closer to calving?' I said quietly, with my back turned to Mrs Pallot in the hope she wouldn't hear the confession of doubt in my own diagnosis.

'Nah, bah cry,' I heard her voice call from behind me. Her hearing aid was hidden away in the upstairs bathroom cabinet of the farmhouse, far away from the auditory canal it was supposed to inhabit, but she was listening in to our every word – proving that perhaps her hearing loss was a little more selective than she'd care to admit after all. 'I've seen cows go down year round!' Mrs Pallot bellowed across at me, rolling the 'r' of 'round' with her strong Jèrriais accent.

'Oh! Is that Mrs Pallot in the background? You'd better tell her she's right!' Greg said down the phone handset. 'Milking Jerseys are more prone so it probably is *still* milk fever even this far after calving,' he said. 'You should have calcium in the visit box – give her a bottle in the vein and she should get up. Start with that anyway and see.'

I thanked him profusely, then apologised, again. And again.

'Right, milk fever. Greg says you're always spot on!' I said, buttering up to Mrs Pallot. I felt a bit sick at myself really, playing along with their decades of flirty banter, but if it won me some brownie points, then so be it.

'Well, Greg knows this place like the back of his hand.' She picked up her walking stick and pointed it at the cow, stabbing the air as she spoke. 'He's fixed more of my girls in the last twenty years than you've had hot dinners. Best vet on the island!'

I retrieved the brown glass bottle of calcium borogluconate from the car, along with a heavy-duty needle and a metre-long rubber pipe with a cupped, bellowed end. There was only one problem. I'd never *actually* given a cow a bottle of calcium on my own before. 'Shall we have a go then?' I said, feigning confidence to Mrs Pallot.

I took wide strides over the straw bedding to reach the cow. There was a bucket of untouched cattle feed and a separate bucket of water by her head, neither of any interest to the cow. I knelt in the straw next to her head and ran my hand over the velvet smooth hair of her long, swerved neck. I uncapped the large gauged needle and with the other hand, attempted to occlude and raise the cow's jugular vein. As I knelt there beside the recumbent beast, I raised the vein, but the cow swerved her head outwards and in front of her, and knocked both my hands way off target. I tried again, but each time I lined up, she threw her head at the very last minute in her last-ditch tactical attempt to bat me away just before I could actually place the needle.

In my mind, I think of Jersey cows as being quite placid

animals, with their doe-eyed faces, pastel caramel-coloured hides and long, blinking eyelashes. And for the large part they are (except the bulls!). But that doesn't make them on a par with a domesticated animal. Asking any unrestrained dog, cat or horse to remain completely still for an intravenous injection would be a tall order. So, to expect that of a farm animal was utterly naive of me.

'Just . . . throw it in the vein there . . . see it . . . right there,' Mrs Pallot said, standing on the sidelines watching my every move.

Yep, that is exactly what I'm trying to do! I thought to myself as the cow headbutted my hand away once more. 'Do you have a head rope? Or anything we could use to try and keep her head a little stable?'

'A head rope? No, no, no! Greg's never needed a head rope!' she replied. 'You just need to get it into the vein, *there.*' She pointed again with her stick at the cow's neck.

What I'd really hoped for (and perhaps expected) was a 'cattle crush' – which sounds a lot scarier than it is. Many farms will have a metal cage that can act like stocks, restraining an animal for treatment and making it safer for both the veterinary staff and the animal. Through all our veterinary training, our cattle patients were always presented safely restrained, yet here the cow was free, loose and able to run, charge or bolt at me (or worse, Mrs Pallot). There was no cattle crush on the farm. The only other option would be to ask for one more pair of hands to come and take hold of the bowling ball of a head by placing a thumb and forefinger into the nostrils of the cow, so the head could be temporarily restrained just long enough for me to place the line. But asking a pensioner to come and kneel in the straw bed, restrain the head of a cow and not get hurt while doing so just somehow felt a little risky.

So I tried again, and the cow jolted its head once more. I dropped the needle. I started again. I occluded the vein, lined up the needle, went to push it through the skin, but as soon as the cow felt the sharp stab of the metal needle point, she swung her head and knocked me out of position. *Damn.*

I tried manually swinging her head to the left, then pushed my back against her muzzle and attempted to insert the needle that way, with my contorted body angled away from her. That time, I managed to insert the needle through the skin, but I was way off target. I pulled out slightly, re-angled the needle and then re-advanced it deeper into the cow's neck. Then BINGO.

'OK, I'm in.' A slow trickle of red blood dripped through the needle hub. I reached to grasp hold of the calcium bottle. In and amongst all the kerfuffle, it had moved out of my arm's reach. Mrs Pallot started hobbling over. 'Thank you!' I said to her as she managed to bend down with remarkable ease, lift the bottle and hand it to me.

But as I attempted to connect the bottle and rubber tubing to the end of the needle, the cow panicked. Possibly aware that two humans had now entered the space in which she had chosen to recline. In a mad dash attempt to escape, she hurled her body forwards, her front legs swung out from underneath her and her chest rose off the straw bed. She was still too weak to stand fully, but instead had managed to elevate herself up into a 'dog sitting' position.

Of course, the many kilograms of a cow's body against that of one new grad vet is never a fair arm wrestle. And so, as she swung her body forwards, she pushed her head firmly against my back, making me stumble forwards, and, of course, I lost my balance. Not only did I stumble, though, I also dropped the precious (and only) bottle of calcium. In doing so, because the bottle was connected to the tube, which was in turn connected to the perfectly placed needle sitting in the cow's jugular vein, everything came flying with it.

I dived for the calcium bottle, in a similar fashion to the moment in a film where some precious treasure is hurled into the air and someone leaps with outstretched arms in slow motion to stop it from falling onto the ground and smashing. But sadly, unlike in the movies, the bottle fell right through my freezing cold fingers and plopped straight down into a well-trodden yet still pretty fresh cowpat. I retrieved the bottle from the brown sloppy mess on the barn floor, and held it up to the flickering dim light to see if there was any hope of salvation – only to spot two strands of straw bedding floating slowly around the liquid inside. I hung my head in disappointment and wanted to scream the loudest profanity I could. Cows *are* pretty amazing healers. But even for a cow, to receive unfiltered, faecally contaminated liquid calcium directly into the vein would have been a slow, septic death sentence.

I had no choice but to make another phone call back to the practice.

I cannot begin to describe the incompetence I felt at having to ask Greg to come and take over. He was on call, which was the only saving grace to my otherwise hideously low self-esteem at that point. He was also the more laissez-faire of the various partners in the practice – which helped. But as I had no more calcium in the car, he told me to stay put and he'd come and meet me there.

Greg arrived. I walked to the car and began apologising profusely. I recalled where we had got to and apologised again for how inept I felt. Greg just laughed through a tobacco-infused cough, and told me to 'chill', being the ex-surfer type with a pretty relaxed approach to most things in life. We both stepped back into the barn and Mrs Pallot's face lit up at the sight of Greg. The cow had reclined back into her recumbent position, her neck shaped like a hook as she looked behind herself once again.

Greg calmy walked up to the cow, stroked her neck, swiftly placed a needle into the vein, connected the rubber tubing, held the bottle of calcium above his head, and patiently waited while the calcium trickled steadily into the cow's circulatory system without her even moving a muscle.

Are you flippin' kidding me? were the words in my head.

The cow simply lay there and held her neck beautifully still as Greg administered the life-saving fresh bottle of *sterile* calcium into her body. I'm convinced she even moo'd a 'thank you' to Greg as soon as he stood back up.

'There we go,' Greg said, as he withdrew the needle and folded the rubber tubing neatly and proficiently around his hand. It was clear he had done this a thousand times. It was also clear that despite having completed my degree, I still had so, so much learning left to do.

On the drive home from the farm that night I had a flashback to the moment I graduated – the exhilaration and excitement I felt that I could finally begin living the dream; how I was filled to the brim with confidence. I was ecstatic. I'd seen an advert for a practice on Jersey looking for a new graduate vet and I was up for the adventure. The Channel Islands, even now, ignite a flame within me. They were a place I felt connected to and somewhere I could very easily call home, having visited many times as a Gerald Durrell-obsessed child. And so, I did. A few months into practice, though, I can remember asking myself where my feelings of confidence and self-belief had disappeared to? What practice life had taught me, very early on, was just how wide the gap was between my theoretical knowledge and my practical skills.

I *knew* Mrs Pallot's cow needed a bottle of calcium. OK, I needed some reassurance that I was on the right track with the diagnosis, but the stumbling block was not the theoretical but the practical. The 'how to' of it all. I can remember looking at that bottle of calcium and thinking, *I know I need you to get into that cow's vein. But I beg of you, please, just someone show me how?*

It was hard not to feel somewhat debilitated, by not having sufficient practical skills to put my knowledge to proper use. We all got taught the theory, but the majority of practical skills were picked up or taught in private practice. Nothing formal, it was down to each practice to decide how much (or little) time they would invest in training up a veterinary student on placement or a new graduate vet in practice. Which meant each new grad had a widely varied, individual experience when it came to how fast they would progress out in the 'real world' of veterinary medicine.

I'll never forget the eye roll of a colleague as I walked into the prep area. She was trying to unblock a male cat under sedation. This is where a catheter is passed up a male cat's urethra that has occluded, usually caused by a small stone, a mucus plug or a muscular spasm. Either way, if the pipework stays blocked, the bladder reaches bursting point which can sadly lead to death. A 'blocked cat' is always treated as an emergency.

The idea is to try to flush past the blockage with the catheter, but this in itself is not always as easy as it sounds. As I walked into the room, she asked if I had ever unblocked a cat, to which *obviously* I had no choice but to say no. 'Of course you haven't,' she muttered under her breath, then threw the disused catheter into a kidney dish and walked out of the room – oozing with temper and frustration.

I was her second on call, and in hindsight, I don't blame her. She was exhausted and I was useless to her – what was the point of having *me*, as a new graduate, to be *her* second on call? I was no help to her at all. I was probably – if anything – a hindrance. Her pupil, not her peer.

Eventually she gathered herself, deepened the sedation, and managed to pass the catheter. She apologised but those moments of feeling useless stay with you. I didn't blame her, I didn't blame the practice; I blamed myself (perhaps also unfairly) that I could not be of more help and resented my own lack of practical experience.

The one resounding memory from my first year in practice was the constant feeling of teetering on a knife's edge. It felt like an uphill mountain that I had volunteered myself to climb. I questioned *everything*; even the stuff I knew I knew, I'd still question. There is, of course, an ever-present fear of getting struck off if you make a mistake, but focusing even higher than the worry of litigation, just the fact that I had an animal's life in my hands was intensely daunting. I could no longer hide behind being a vet 'in training' – suddenly I *was* the vet. I was accountable. The decisions I made had consequences. This was no longer just theory; this was the real world.

After a few months in practice, the time had come for me to cover my first weekend on call. I didn't sleep a wink for the entire forty-eight hours (mainly because I was in work for the majority of it). As was my nurse, for whom I felt very sorry.

It was manic.

We started with Roger – a huge St Bernard who had torn a flap of skin from his chest. I examined him and found the wound – large enough to fit my fist in – but luckily only skin deep. I anaesthetised him and sutured the wound. It went well. One patient down. Phew. However, as soon as one call was completed, another came in. A cat that had vomited six times. A rabbit that had stopped eating. A horse that had trodden on a nail. A dog that had eaten some chocolate. A cat that had gone lame, followed by a dog that had gone lame, followed by a horse that had gone lame. The calls just kept coming, one after another as a relentless train of sick animals in need of veterinary attention.

More cats, more dogs, more vomit, more diarrhoea, more lameness. Seven vets' worth of work, across three branches, reduced at the weekend to one vet's responsibility. I tried to phone a senior colleague to confess I had eight patients waiting, nothing urgent patient-wise but some very loud 'tuts' and 'sighs' coming from the waiting room full of expectant owners keen for it to be 'their turn next'. I wasn't quite sure how to get through them all, or how I could possibly go any quicker – but with it being eight o'clock on a Saturday night, he encouraged me to just keep going and congratulated me that I was, in his eyes, doing a great job. It was then it dawned on me: *This time round, you're on your own, kid.* There does come a time when you do have to learn to cope

alone, like taking the stabilisers off your bike or the armbands off at a swimming class. Maybe this was him handing
me a fairly harsh lesson in resilience training. Regardless,
the potentially catastrophic shit show that it could result in
at the time was a little overwhelming to me if I allowed my
mind to go there, so I just kept plugging away, and focused
instead on whichever job was in hand at the time. I treated
patients one after another, praying that Monday morning
would arrive soon.

Eventually Sunday arrived, and then Sunday afternoon
melted into Sunday evening. I got home and had some tea. I
watched a bit of telly but my mind was elsewhere. All I could
think about was how the weekend had gone. What if I had
got it all wrong? What if I had missed an obvious diagnosis?
What if Roger had a penetrating injury I had missed and I
should have explored deeper? And what if the phone rings
again? Have I got reception? Will I cope? Had I coped? Was
I a shit vet? Catastrophising every scenario had become the
norm.

I had managed to find a flat to rent above a wood carver's
workshop behind Jersey Zoo. Quite fitting to be woken by the
dawn chorus of tropical birds, the sound of howler monkeys
and the golden lion tamarins calling for their morning feed
– as opposed to backfiring car engines and drunken Saturday
night revellers knocking on the front door of the temporary
flat I had moved in to on arrival to the island, located right
in the centre of town.

I had fallen asleep in front of the telly and was rudely
awoken by the 'on call vet's' mobile phone, flashing and
ringing as it slid down the curve of the sofa arm, like a kid
riding on a park slide, and clonked me on the forehead. It

was another call. 5.14 a.m. Although this time, it was from one of the nurses in the practice.

'Hello, Cathy?'

'Hi, James, I'm really sorry to phone, but I'm really worried about Beth.'

Beth was her smooth-coated Hungarian vizsla, a completely delightful canine companion. Tall, slender with a stunning coat the colour of a gingernut biscuit from nose to tail. She was friendly. She pushed her muzzle into my leg to encourage a gentle pat on her head and would nudge me for another as soon as I tried to pull my hand away. I had met her a few times at the practice as she had been in for some ultrasound scans. Not because she was ill – quite the opposite. She was a perfectly healthy two-year-old, in fine fettle. But Beth was carrying some very precious cargo – she was pregnant – and she had been due to whelp any day.

'OK, what's happened?'

For Cathy to phone *me*, I knew something must be of real concern. Cathy had bred many litters before; she was experienced. She had seen and done it all.

She began to explain that she had seen Beth go into first-stage labour earlier on Sunday afternoon. Her body temperature had dropped the day before, indicating that labour was imminent. First-stage labour can last for many hours for dogs, so that wasn't necessarily unusual. The unusual part was that as she progressed to second-stage labour, and after a couple of early contractions, no puppy had appeared. Instead, Beth had stopped straining and had started to wander around the living room.

'OK,' I said, trying to desperately rattle my brain through the dystocia section of my reproduction notes from uni. 'Have you seen any green discharge or blood coming from her?'

'No, there's been nothing.'

'OK. Erm . . .'

Cathy interjected, 'Do you mind coming out? I think she may need some oxytocin and I don't want to leave her.'

At this stage, I was just grateful for some direction. I agreed, and said I'd be there shortly. On the way I stopped to pick up a bottle of oxytocin (an injection used to exert a contracting effect on the uterus) stored in the refrigerator at the practice and also took the opportunity to flick through my uni notes on 'the whelping bitch'.

As I arrived at the house, Beth was lying down once again and had restarted with some mild contractions. I knelt to smooth my hand along her velvet ginger fur and with her big eyes and drooping ears, she looked up at me and seemed exhausted, as did Cathy, having both stayed up all night trying to interpret Beth's mixed bag of signs.

'I don't know – I just don't like the look of it all,' Cathy said. 'Normally I would have expected the first one to have arrived by now.'

I placed a latex glove on my right hand and squeezed some sterile lubricant jelly across my fingertips and then gently felt as far as I could to see if there was a head or the rump of a stuck puppy in need of retrieval. But there was nothing.

I summarised the options with Cathy, knowing full well that as a vet nurse with twenty years' clinical experience and eight years' breeder experience, she very likely already *knew* her options. But she humoured me at least and allowed me some time to gather my thoughts.

'We could try oxytocin to help her contractions, but if she's pushing against a puppy that is physically stuck, it's not without risk to her or her puppies,' was my first offering.

'Or I could take a blood sample and drive it to the practice to check her calcium levels, but that's going to take an hour or so at least, so it might be quicker to take her in and then we can start treatment if we need to.' My second.

'I really don't want to have to take her into work,' Cathy said, hoping our luck may still turn.

'Or we could go straight for a caesarean section, given the timings and her unproductive straining.' I threw out my third offering.

A bold offering, as I had absolutely no idea how to perform the caesarean surgery on my own. I had only spayed two bitches by that point; both operations had gone very well but had also been under the gloved guidance of a more senior vet.

I was also really, *really* hoping our luck might turn.

'OK, let's go for the oxytocin first,' Cathy requested.

Fine. I drew up a dose of oxytocin into a syringe and then injected it into Beth's back muscle. She didn't seem to flinch as her mind was focused on other more pressing matters.

We agreed to give Beth some time. We made a cup of tea and watched her from a distance, hoping that her contractions might restart, and she would produce a puppy.

Please, please produce a puppy.

The time ticked by. Ten minutes felt like an hour, and still, no puppy. After another ten minutes, a few more contractions but *still* no puppy. Onto a second cup of tea and we reviewed the options once more. I had another feel of Beth, but there was *still no puppy* in the birth canal.

By then, I really was beginning to worry. It had been a good hour since Cathy had first made the telephone call.

'Can we give a second oxytocin?' Cathy asked.

'Well, we *can* . . . but I'm just really worried as to why she's not produced anything yet.' I looked over at Cathy. 'I *do* think we need to start considering whether she needs a caesarean.'

Cathy looked understandably concerned. A caesarean section would mean taking Beth into surgery, which is not without risk, even in the hands of an experienced surgeon. Having said that, if we left it too late, and each subsequent puppy started to separate from their own individual placenta with no way of exiting the womb, they would suffocate inside her. Risk was involved whichever way we played it. Taking any pregnant dog to surgery is a judgement call between the risk to dog versus the risk to the puppies – a judgement call I had *never* had to make on my own back and for which I felt woefully inadequate. Although my gut instinct was telling me, if not screaming at me, that I should get Beth to the practice pronto.

'Can we give her one more oxytocin?' Cathy said, defiantly.

Cathy was known in the practice to be quite a force to reckon with. I could appreciate that she desperately wanted to avoid surgery, but it made me uncomfortable that we were about to delay even further. 'OK. Well, let's give one more oxytocin,' I replied, 'but if this doesn't work, we *really* need to think about plan B.'

After a further fifteen minutes, still no puppies had arrived. Beth was lying in her bed on her side with her head lolloping over the cushioned edge. Her contractions were increasingly spaced. Nothing was happening.

'I'm going to call Chris,' I said. I needed a second opinion. The tension over whether to take her to surgery or not had built – and it felt beyond my judgement call. Chris was the senior surgeon in the practice, well trusted by staff and clients as the 'go-to' for a definitive opinion. It was 6.30 a.m., not too ridiculously early, but still my heart pounded with nerves as the telephone rang, unsure of what sort of reception I might be letting myself in for.

'Hi, Chris, it's James. I'm so sorry to phone.'

He dismissed my apology immediately and asked how he could help. He was probably about seven or eight years ahead of me. My palpating heart calmed as soon as I realised he wasn't too pissed off with my early Monday morning advice request. I explained the situation.

'James, you need to take her to surgery ASAP,' Chris summarised without any hesitation.

'Where are you now?'

'I'm with Cathy. Err, sorry, I'm at her house.' I was nervous; my words stumbled. I'd needed his help more now than ever, but should I ask him to come in or would I be expected to try to sort this on my own?

'Is she there? Can you put her on for me?'

I handed the phone to Cathy. She paced around the room, recounting Beth's behaviour over the past twenty-four hours. There was a lot of 'yep', 'uh-huh', 'yep' sounds. Then finally a resounding 'OK'.

She handed the phone back to me. 'Hi, mate. OK, you need to get straight to the practice. Cathy'll bring Beth. Josie will already be sorting in-patients so she can do the anaesthetic with you. Get a cannula into Beth, don't give any pre-med, just propofol off the needle – you'll need to take the dose up a bit – around six mils per kilo. Start prepping her and I'll get there as soon as I can.'

74

The relief.

'Yep, OK,' I replied and was about to hang up before Chris continued, 'James, JAMES?'

'Yeah?'

'If I'm not there before you're ready to open her up, then go ahead and start – we need to be quick. Just make the incision as you would for a spay, like we did the other day. Pack around the uterus with ex lap swabs, carefully incise into it and milk each puppy down in turn. You'll be fine. Just hand Josie or Cathy each pup and you stay focused on Beth. OK?'

Shit. 'Err, yep. OK.' My heart was pounding once again.

'Thank you!'

I hung up. *Shit, shit, SHIT*, I said silently in my own head.

Cathy was already encouraging Beth out of her bed to start getting her into the car. 'You go ahead and start getting everything ready with Josie and I'll be a few minutes behind,' she called across the living room to me.

I hurried to the car and put my foot down. Moments later we were in the more familiar surroundings of the clinical environment. There was something reassuring about being surrounded by the drugs, the tools, the team, the equipment that enables a vet to perform as a vet. With Josie, Cathy placed the cannula into Beth's foreleg, while I started collecting together the scrub kit, surgical gown, hat, gloves, mask and suture material that I would need for the caesarean surgery. After twenty minutes or so, everything was set. We were ready to go. But there was no sign of Chris.

'Shall I start?' I asked Cathy. 'Or would you rather wait? I won't be offended.'

Cathy took a moment to consider the options.

'Start,' she replied confidently. 'I'd like you to start. I just wanna get the puppies out now.'

I gave a defiant nod in return; we were all in agreement. I would start the surgery. I plunged the chalky white propofol anaesthetic agent through the cannula in Beth's vein and watched her slowly drift into unconsciousness. A tap on the eyelid confirmed she was asleep. Josie lifted her head. Her jaw relaxed. I pulled forwards her tongue and placed the breathing tube down into her windpipe. Once she was asleep and the anaesthetic was stable, we rolled her onto her back, clipped the fur from her belly and the nurses began to sterilise the skin. I asked the two nurses if they were happy for me to start scrubbing or whether to wait and help them transfer the forty-odd kilograms of vizsla through to the theatre (also hoping it might buy me a bit of justified extra time for Chris to arrive).

'You start scrubbing, we'll lift her.'

I tried to remain calm (and appear calm), stay focused, but underneath I was praying that Chris would burst through the practice doors at any moment. All the while, the voice in my head just kept repeating the panicked profanities.

I was gowned and sterile, with an instrument tray to my side and Beth positioned on the operating table. I placed four large paper drapes across her body, leaving a sterile window along her midline. No more procrastinating. No more playing for extra time. I picked up the scalpel, and with Josie monitoring the anaesthetic, I started to swipe the scalpel blade along the skin of Beth's abdomen.

I passed through skin, then subcutaneous white fat, and eventually to the white line of the linea alba – recognised as the meeting point of the abdominal muscles along her underside. My hands were shaking. Each step I carefully navigated using a combination of the scalpel, scissors and forceps. Then lastly, I picked up the muscle layer with my forceps and made a stab incision through to the abdominal cavity.

Where the hell is Chris? I thought to myself. My mouth was dry and my heart raced.

As I extended my incision further forwards, sitting just beneath the muscle, the huge gravid uterus filled the abdominal cavity. I reached both hands into the abdomen and started to pull the swollen, pale pink uterus forwards when suddenly the operating doors to the theatre flung open and Chris burst through. He was already gowned and pulling on a pair of surgical gloves. 'Oh, Jeez! Sorry, that took me a while,' he spluttered out the words. He was out of breath, panting like a dog – his cheeks glowed bright red, just visible above his surgeon's mask. He looked like he was about to pass out.

'Are you OK?' I asked.

'Wife's got the car, taken the kids to nursery.' He stood up, arched his back slightly and took in a massive deep inhalation of air into his lungs. 'So I ran here!'

'Oh my God,' Cathy replied. 'Thank you,' she said, acknowledging his commitment to help out his colleagues and a very pregnant Beth.

'OK . . . how far have you got?' he asked between his deep inhalations.

'I've just reached the uterus,' I said, handing the forceps and scalpel over Beth's body towards Chris.

'What are you handing me those for?' he asked, still panting. 'This is your surgery.'

77

He took another deep inhale then swallowed hard and continued. 'So next you need to pack around the abdomen with your swabs and then make your incision to the uterus just ... about ... there.' He pointed with his index finger over the fleshy pink wrinkled surface of the uterine body.

I smiled behind my mask and picked up the scalpel.

If you imagine the uterus is shaped like a 'Y', I was making my incision over the stalk, rather than either of the two arms. The walls of the uterus peeled apart from each other and just through the opening, I could see a dark brown circular 'blob' – a similar colour to Beth's chestnut coat – suspended in a transparent sack of watery clear fluid.

'OK.' I looked up at Chris, who had by now managed to correct his own oxygen saturation levels.

'Right, so now you need to incise into the amniotic sack and then retrieve the puppy.'

I picked up the scalpel once again and carefully 'popped' the water balloon. Clear fluid erupted from the incision site as I reached in to feel for the foetus. I tried to take hold of the puppy, but it was surprisingly slippery. I used my fingers to grab around his body, like the metal claw of an arcade game trying to retrieve a cuddly toy by the seaside, then once I'd worked out my grip, I pulled the puppy from the warm pool within the uterus to the oxygenated air of the outside world.

'Great!' Chris called out. 'OK, right, let's clamp the umbilicus. I normally put two clamps, so one here ...' Chris reached over and applied an artery forcep to the cord, clamping the vessels shut between the jarred teeth of the instrument. 'And then one just below, about here.' He applied a second artery forcep. 'And then use your scissors to cut between the two clamps.'

With the puppy suspended in my left hand, I sliced through the rubbery umbilical cord and the puppy was free.

'So drop him into the towel, but don't touch anything as you need to stay sterile, James. Cathy will catch the puppy.'

Cathy was standing with her hands holding out an opened towel like a sling. I dropped the puppy into her makeshift hammock, and she began rubbing vigorously on his sides, willing and wishing him to take a first breath.

'Well done. Now we need to really gently put some tension on the other artery forcep and slowly, slowly tease the placenta from the uterine wall.'

I picked up the two handles of the instrument and very gently pulled with just enough force to feel the tiniest bit of give as the placenta peeled away from the uterus. As I did so, I looked over at the first puppy in Cathy's hands. It was still motionless.

'OK, James? Stay focused. So now you just keep going!' Chris interrupted my wandering attention as Cathy left the theatre with the puppy.

I milked the second puppy down and followed the same procedure. She was smaller, much smaller than the first. And wriggled as soon as I freed her from her sac. I dropped her into Josie's towelled hands this time, who also began the vigorous rubbing. Within seconds of being born, the puppy started squeaking and lifting its head. The third puppy of similar frame to the second soon followed. And the fourth. Meanwhile, I noticed Cathy had taken the first puppy through to the prep area and was assembling a second anaesthetic machine to start delivering oxygen.

By then a couple more nurses had arrived who all picked

up towels and hovered by the theatre doors awaiting to be handed a puppy. Five, six, seven.

'How's the first pup doing?' I called through the theatre doors, but Cathy had a stethoscope in her ears and her back to me, still focused on the little one's revival. There was no answer.

I asked one of the nurses standing by the theatre doors if there was an update. 'He's not there yet,' she said, holding and rubbing puppy number seven in her towel, 'but I think Cathy said there is still a heartbeat and he's on oxygen so they're still trying.'

Four nurses stood eagerly poised and ready as they each rubbed the newborn puppies when they arrived. We set up a carrier crate with a heated blanket so as the revived puppies were strong enough, they could move into their own blanketed safe space.

Eight, nine, ten puppies.

The chaos was immense, yet all I could hear were the cheers of nurses as each subsequent puppy took their first breath in response to all the towel rubbing that woke them up from their snoozing amniotic dreams.

And still they came, eleven, twelve. Yet, no news on the first puppy.

The other eleven puppies were all doing great. But the tension surrounding Cathy in the prep area was palpable. Did she need any help? Did she *want* any help? Or did she want to be left to call the shots by herself. Did she blame me? Should I have done something differently? Perhaps I should have phoned Chris sooner? Perhaps I should not have given the second oxytocin injection. Was this all my fault?

Suddenly, 'That was a breath!' I heard the student nurse

Vicky call across the prep room. She flung her arm out and pointed at the motionless puppy on the table. 'I swear that was a breath!'

Then the sound of a huge cheer from the whole nursing team. The puppy had *finally* taken a first breath, all of its own accord. I saw Cathy drop her shoulders and heave a sigh of relief.

And still, there was one more to come. Thirteen was the final puppy count. Thirteen puppies in total.

Chris talked me through suturing closed the uterine body, then the muscle, and then the skin. Finally, Josie switched off the anaesthetic gas and maintained Beth on pure oxygen to aid her recovery.

'Well, I think we've just created a whole load of work for you here, Cathy!' Chris winked at me and called from the theatre to the prep area. 'I hope you weren't planning on going on holiday for the next few weeks!'

I didn't, but there was definitely a moment there when I could have cried with relief that, for my part at least, it was all over. I was physically, emotionally, mentally drained and exhausted. The theatre resembled a crime scene – bloody towels strewn across the floor, the sodden drapes that once had kept Beth's surgical site sterile now screwed up on the operating table, the anaesthetic machine abandoned with needle caps, used syringes and pipework left dangling. The surgical table, at exactly waist height, had allowed the blood and birthing fluids to seep through my surgical gown, then my scrubs, and it continued all the way through to my boxer shorts from leaning over Beth's surgery. I was a mess – and still had a full day of work ahead of me. I wouldn't be home again until seven o'clock that evening and with no change of clothes, it was going to be a long (and soggy!) day ahead.

We de-gowned and I helped carry Beth through to a comfy bed to recover. Her head sleepily lolled around as we shuffled her across the prep room. On the way back to have a look at the puppies, I felt Chris tap me on the back. 'That's your first caesarean done, mate. Well done, you smashed it! That's another one you can tick off the list.'

I thanked him. Thanked him over and over. I can't put into words the gratitude I felt. Importantly, all the puppies were fine, even the first huge bruiser of a puppy that was blocking the road for his siblings. And Beth made a speedy recovery.

I learnt so much that day. And with a vet like Chris, I knew I had found a true mentor. The early experiences as a graduate vet are incredibly formative. Having heard the disappointment and disillusionment coming from some friends at the time, who felt let down by their unsupportive first jobs and were questioning their ability or desire to stay working in clinical practice, I knew without a doubt that I had landed on my feet having found such a brilliant team in Jersey. I was one of the lucky ones. And for that, I will be eternally grateful.

CHAPTER 5

Rocky

Ms Jeffries, in her mid to late sixties, answered the door to her one-bedroom flat wearing only a pale pink silk dressing gown, tied at the waist, with a matching silk eye mask pulled onto her head and resting neatly upon her greyish-blue wispy, bouffant hair. The sound of tinkling classical music played somewhere in the distance. A sweet, potent aroma hit me as I stepped into her hallway – a combination of the five or six white plastic triangular air fresheners she had picked up from the one-pound bargain shop and the heavy dose of her rose-scented perfume she had perhaps applied at the sound of the doorbell.

She had bright blue eye shadow painted across her upper eyelids, and a thick layer of white Oil of Olay cream plastered across her cheeks with a further strip across her forehead. It was like being greeted by Mrs Doubtfire and the infamous scene right after she plunges her whole face into the white frosting of a huge cake. I could be excused for thinking I'd interrupted a mid-afternoon home spa session, and the very first time I turned up, that was my exact presumption. However, this was the fifth home visit to Ms Jeffries' flat and I soon realised this was just how Ms Jeffries chose to spend a normal day – caked in anti-wrinkle cream, listening to music and sipping sherry, which she would insist I should at least have a small drop of before I went back to continue my consults in the afternoon.

I liked her. She was kind, harmless and extraordinarily flamboyant. The first of many wonderfully eccentric people I would go on to meet through my veterinary career and also the first client who had requested me by name as her preferred vet, for which I was delighted – as it gave me the excuse to leave the confines of my consulting room and pay her another visit that afternoon.

Standing in the living room, Ms Jeffries was demonstrating to me the action of her four-year-old female tortoiseshell cat called Gabriella, who had developed another bout of kitty cystitis, a condition often linked to stress. A cat so nervous, she couldn't even face going to the loo. Ms Jeffries crossed the two panels of her silk dressing gown with her arms and tucked them between her legs. Then she rotated ninety degrees and with a slight bend of her knees, she leant slightly forwards and dropped into a squat position. She then stood up straight and turned to face me briefly before she rotated once more and bent back down into another squat. This was her doing what she had titled Gabriella's 'turn and squat', and the charade usually went on for at least a minute.

'She went turn ... and then squat ... Turn ... and squat ... Turn, squat.'

I watched, applauded and thanked her for her most excellent impression. After I politely declined the drop of sherry, she told me to head into the bedroom to seek out Gabriella. I lifted one edge of the pale blue eiderdown fitted neatly over her double bed, and revealed the big wide yellow eyes of a cat who looked both petrified and pained. A cursory exam revealed nothing abnormal and so, once again, I left copious amounts of pain relief and spent the next twenty minutes discussing with Ms Jeffries how we could make her flat a little more feline friendly and a few tips on how we might reduce some of the mental health stresses that Gabriella was struggling with, leading her to another bout of cystitis. One likely factor being Ms Jeffries' constant endeavour to follow her cat around the small flat while clutching a bottle of Dettol antibacterial spray, ready to give a quick spritz to any urine spots that may otherwise have gone unnoticed.

'Well, I've got to watch her or she'll do it annnnnywhere,' she said in her camp, overexaggerated way. I tried to explain, again, that this was perhaps quite a strong contributing factor to the cause of the problem – that poor Gabriella probably felt it was quite unnerving, being chased by a giant bottle of Dettol – but I feared, once again, that it would fall on deaf ears.

So I left her with some non-absorbent litter in an attempt to collect a sample and suggested she bought a few more litter trays, as a compromise, in the hope it might encourage Gabriella to be a little more considerate in her choice of lavatory location but on the proviso that Ms Jeffries must also keep her side of the bargain and give her poor cat a little privacy.

Having the chance to observe and then examine cats in their 'home' environment often gives me a much greater insight into their wellbeing and perhaps enables a more holistic approach to their veterinary care as cats are, to some extent, extraordinarily private and complex animals. The environment or home they live in can be hugely influential in not only their mental health, but it can impact their physical health too. When at the vet's, it's not unusual for an examination to be a little unrewarding. Often, cats just don't give very much away.

Which is perhaps not so surprising when you consider the mechanics of a trip to the vet's for a cat. They arrive at the practice, often after losing a battle of wills at home to avoid stepping their paws into the dreaded cat carrier. Then they get driven in a car (or wheeled along in a pram, as in Ms Jeffries' case), something dogs perhaps grow accustomed to, but must be so scary for a cat. And then, they find themselves placed onto my consulting-room table. Thankfully, 'scruffing' cats has now been recognised by most as an unnecessary and painful way to handle our feline friends. But asking a cat to voluntarily leave the safety of their cat carrier and engage in an examination is often harder than it may seem. Many will freeze at the very back of their cocooned safe haven, despite offering them some treats. Some are even able to withstand a gentle tilt, and some can even defy gravity altogether and use all four feet to bridge across the door opening with the cat carrier upended and hovering perpendicular to the table. I always feel a sense of relief (and this is perhaps a cheeky request to all cat owners) when an owner turns up with a cat carrier with an easily removable lid.

Once I have managed to extract the poor feline lurking within their crate, most cats do tolerate a clinical examination pretty well. I say tolerate, as often the adrenaline kicks in and they wait for the ordeal to be over and done with. Often owners will hand out such praise as 'oooph, he wouldn't let me do that at home!' as my fingertips prise open the jaws of the family 'tiger', booked in under an owner complaint of 'smelly breath'. Or, of course, there is the magic 'disappearing lameness' – a limping cat at home will often strut around the consulting room quite happily, perfectly sound. They'll even jump off the table if they so wish – to the gasps and disbelief of the disgruntled owner who concludes that their moggy has just mugged them off by insisting on a forty-quid bill at the vet's for me to confirm to them that their cat seems in fine health. Of course, it's often the adrenaline of the visit that masks the pain, but I like to imagine the cat sitting in the carrier filing their nails, listening in and nodding along to all the compliments I'm paying them as I hand over a bottle of pain relief to owner.

It just seems a thing that most cats can and do behave very differently at the vet's, especially at the end of the consult and the reappearance of the afore-loathed cat carrier. The owners stand with a face of utter incomprehension as the same cat that had only forty minutes previously fought tooth and nail to avoid stepping foot in the dreaded cat carrier at home just voluntarily darts straight back inside in front of the vet. Magic sorcerers we are not. It is merely a sign of the intelligence of a cat. Perhaps they recognise that clambering into the carrier means they'll soon likely be transported back to the safe familiarity of their home environment: their own smells, their own routine, their own company.

'He's just not quite right,' said Emily, a busy mum who had made an emergency appointment that morning, having come straight from the kids' drop-off at school. I'd met Rocky a few weeks previously; he had been in for his third annual vaccination. He was a chunky British Blue pedigree cat, whose lovely smooth thick coat was the colour of gun-metal grey from nose to tail, with two huge golden eyes that looked like solidified marbles of fossilised amber, encased around jet-black pupils. At his vaccination appointment, he didn't appreciate being overly fussed, but seemed fairly happy with the prospect of my hand running down his spine as he arched his back and lifted his tail high into the air. But that was then, and this was a new day, and a very different cat had arrived.

'He's not eaten now for a couple of days,' Emily informed me as she pulled a long knitting needle through the white plastic-coated metal hoops of Rocky's wire carrier, having lost the original metal rod the basket came with. She placed the knitting needle to one side, lifted the lid of the carrier and looked at me expectantly.

'I don't know what it is. I can't quite put my finger on it, but just *something* about him isn't right,' she reiterated.

Had there been any changes to his drinking or urinating habits, had he suffered with any diarrhoea, or had she seen him vomit? I asked. But as is often the case, my enquiry was met with an apologetic shrug of her shoulders.

'He spends most of his time outside, if I'm honest. I couldn't rule it out, I s'pose? But I've not seen anything around the house.'

I could tell she was concerned. Rocky normally followed a fairly predictable routine but for him to refuse his morning breakfast altogether was pretty unheard of.

'OK, let's take a look at him.'

After a few introductory chin rubs, I reached in to lift Rocky out of his carrier. His front nails tangled into the cotton loops of the pale blue towel he had arrived on, Emily reached forwards to unclip them as I held Rocky suspended in the air, then once freed, I lowered him onto my consulting-room table.

He crouched into a low sitting position and held his ears slightly back, an expression to suggest he would tolerate this but I shouldn't go as far as to suggest he was enjoying the experience, by any measure.

He allowed me to check his gum colour, which was a salmon pink and had a slimy, hydrated appearance. His eyes were bright, there was no coughing, no heart murmur, no scuffed nails (a tell-tale sign of whether a cat has been hit by a car, as they grip to the tarmac road) and his femoral pulses were both present and throbbing at the same time and rate as his heartbeat.

I attempted a temperature reading. Emily held on to Rocky's shoulders while I gently lifted his tail and inserted the metal tip of a digital thermometer. It beeped at 39.1 degrees centigrade. Normal.

I pinched the skin over his spine and carefully pulled it away from the muscle layer underneath, then released my fingers and the skin sprang immediately back to its original position, a rudimentary test to indicate his hydration status. Also normal.

'Well, he's not really giving me much so far,' I informed Emily. 'Everything seems pretty good.'

'He's definitely not right,' she said defiantly, as though I was beginning to question her instincts and she was beginning to question my detective skills.

'No, no, I agree.' I quickly confirmed my allegiance.

I gently encouraged Rocky into 'standing position' and

asked Emily to steady his front end while I had a good feel of his abdomen.

He gave a low-pitch grumble as we lifted his body, a warning perhaps that he was growing impatient of the examination as I gently felt around the front section of his tummy.

'It's OK,' Emily reassured him with a stroke over his head, then she looked up at me. 'That's a bit unusual for him,' in reference to the growly grumble noise he had just offered up.

Then, as I moved my two hands a little further back towards his hips, Rocky suddenly let out a loud 'REEEAAAOOOOW-WWWW' and turned his head and stared directly at my hand, then 'KHHLLLAAAAAA' he hissed loudly. Emily pulled her hands away as Rocky seemed to transform into an entirely different personality. I too pulled my hands away, but the movement seemed to trigger Rocky even more. He kept his body low to the table, pulled his ears back flat against his head and with a rapid swipe of his right foreleg, his claws met the back of my hand. He hissed once more, then spotted an opportunity. Having warned us both off, Rocky darted towards the edge of my consulting-room table and with a new found athleticism he leapt from my table to the floor, then straight up and onto my cupboard work surface.

He clattered past a Perspex unit that displayed a selection of promotional leaflets, which then knocked into a metal pen pot. The Perspex filing unit toppled, as the rest of his body continued to scramble through the maze of stationary, knocking over the cold cup of tea I hadn't quite managed to finish since our receptionist had kindly delivered it at the start of consults. He was on a mission to find somewhere safe. He continued, leaving behind a path of destruction. The best thing we could do was wait for him to find a spot to settle in, which he eventually did, having clambered across my computer keyboard and lodged himself into the tight corner among the wires and dust behind my computer screen.

'Oh, Rocks,' Emily empathised. 'OK, he's *never* behaved like that.' She looked stunned, worried, shocked.

'I suspect he's in pain,' I suggested, as I ran my bleeding hand under a cold tap and allowed Rocky a moment to gather himself, safely confined behind the computer screen.

I dried my hands and suggested we should conduct some further investigations.

'It seemed around his mid-abdomen that he really flinched,' I began to summarise, 'but I couldn't feel anything specific. To be *that painful*, though? If we don't know when he last peed, it could be that he has a blocked bladder. But it could also be something neuro, or orthopaedic. I can't rule out if there's been an injury, or if he's been knocked by a car. Could be his pancreas? But that would be quite an extreme reaction.' I listed the possible differentials as they came to mind, but really, for him to react so violently, *something* must be seriously wrong.

We agreed that Rocky should be admitted. I hovered his cat carrier near the computer and with a stroke of incredible decency and cooperation, Rocky voluntarily darted back into the safe confines of his towelled carrier, probably under the assumption he'd be going home. For him, though, and me, the day had only just begun.

As I carried Rocky through to the prep area, I began thinking about how to safely approach his care. If he did have a blocked bladder, his kidneys could be under severe strain. If there was a fracture somewhere, I'd need to perform a set of survey radiographs. If he was in severe pain from an inflamed pancreas, I'd need to run some bloodwork. The list went on, but firstly I had to somehow get near him.

With the nursing team holding on to Rocky, wrapped in a towel like a 'kitty burrito', I managed to pass an injection of opiate analgesia mixed with a low dose of some sedative into the muscle of his back. We released him from his towelled embrace, unscathed, and allowed him twenty minutes of peace and quiet, which, if the dose of sedative was sufficient, would hopefully enable him to drift off into a quiet snooze.

Thankfully, it worked.

I returned to the cat ward to find Rocky lying on his bed, with his head resting between his two paws. I lifted him and carried him through to the prep room area. The veterinary nurse placed an oxygen mask over his nose and mouth and applied some lubricant to both of his eyes – it may seem bizarre, but even under heavy sedation, cats rarely close their eyes.

'OK, let's have another feel.'

I palpated once again through the soft insides of Rocky's abdomen to see if I could relocate the pain. I felt around his stomach, I felt both his plum-shaped kidneys, then down to his soft, small bladder only about the size of a grape, which didn't correlate with the hypothesis that he could be blocked, otherwise he would have presented with a taut, full and painful bladder at least the size of an apple.

Without wanting to leave Rocky's side, I asked the nurse to collect together the various components needed to obtain a blood sample, when suddenly, *Woah, what was that?*

I had located something within Rocky's mid-abdomen. Something firm, sitting within an area I would hazard a guess to be his small intestine – firm but only semi solid.

It felt to be almost the length of a wine bottle cork, yet I knew it couldn't be as *surely* there is no way a cat could swallow a wine bottle cork in one – but also, I could squish it. I compressed the mass between my fingers as I continued to palpate and attempt to work out in my mind what it could be I was feeling.

'Perhaps it's just faeces?' I said to Maddy, the nurse helping me that morning, my mouth slightly open as I stared blankly into space, concentrating, trying to solve the puzzle. 'But I can't separate it out or move it along.'

As I continued to manipulate my fingertips around the unknown mystery mass, despite the sedation, Rocky let out a low pitched 'grrrrrrrrrr'. This vocal grumble was the last clue I needed to confirm in my mind that whatever that *something* lodged in his small intestine was, I couldn't ignore it.

'OK.' I stroked along Rocky's back, almost apologising to him that I had just re-triggered his discomfort. 'Let's get an X-ray.'

The nurse, Maddy, lifted Rocky from the table, him draped across her arms like a toy doll, then she lay him on the X-ray table. A couple of moments later, we were gathered around the viewer, able to have a look at Rocky's insides.

The loops of guts looked relatively normal, a map of pale grey pipework that contorted around itself like the complicated and convoluted track lines of a rollercoaster ride. There was no startlingly obvious inanimate object to correlate to whatever it was I had been feeling, and nor were there any particular clues to go on for any other issues to suggest an alternative diagnosis.

It is very unusual to find a foreign body blockage in a cat, as generally speaking, cats are simply far more fastidious than dogs! But my suspicions with Rocky were high. After a long discussion, we agreed the most sensible next step would be to perform an exploratory laparotomy, which is a fancy way of saying, 'Let's open him up, and find out.' There was a risk we may have found nothing, that the offending mass could just be a nugget of softer faeces, trying to work its way through Rocky's digestive system, but my instincts were telling me not to leave it to chance.

I phoned Emily. She agreed and requested that I should proceed to take Rocky to surgery.

With Rocky fully anaesthetised, and lying on his back, his belly shaved of fur and skin sterilised with an iodine scrub, it was time to find out what it was that I had felt.

With the bleeping anaesthetic machine in the background, and my usual attire of surgical gloves, a pale blue paper sterile gown, a hair net that made me look like I should work in a bakery and a hot, cotton fabric mask covering my nose and mouth, I began my incision.

My scalpel blade skated along the skin and subcutaneous tissues, then through and into the abdominal cavity. First, I had to get my bearings. Starting at the 'front end', I located Rocky's liver, had a look at his pancreas and then I was able to locate the first section of his small intestine at the exit point of his stomach. The small intestine is coloured rose pink, an elongated pipeline that usually sits flattened when empty, as opposed to circular. If you imagine a well-cooked tube of penne pasta, a metre long, which could flatten or expand with each nugget of faeces that passed through, that is how it felt as I ran the full length of the gastrointestinal tract between my gently pinched thumb and forefinger, checking to feel for any obstructions.

With the nursing team watching, anticipating, and willing me to discover 'something' to explain Rocky's presenting signs, it is always an anxious start. There is a chance with an exploratory laparotomy that we may not discover anything unusual, which is disappointing but not an entirely useless finding – ruling out is often as useful as ruling in when working out a diagnosis. An exploratory laparotomy is, after all, just another diagnostic step, even though the procedure is surgical. Though, having to phone an owner and explain the findings were unremarkable is always a tricky conversation to have, to temper their disappointment while still having to charge for something that I understand may, with hindsight, feel like an 'unnecessary' procedure.

However, in Rocky, something had been found.

'Ahhhh, here it is,' I confirmed to Maddy, who had handed over the anaesthetic duties to a colleague so she could scrub in to help with the surgery. Something was lurking within the tube of corresponding small intestine, which had in turn changed from a rose pink to a muddy maroon colour.

I lifted the portion of impacted gut up and away from the abdomen itself, to exteriorise my target, and then packed some moistened swabs into and around the abdominal cavity. The main risk here would be of contamination. Even though the intestines were empty, with Rocky having not eaten a full meal for almost forty-eight hours, there would still be some liquid intestinal contents. As soon as I cut into the portion of gut, if those digestive liquids dripped or seeped into the abdominal cavity, it could trigger a septic peritonitis, an infection of the abdominal cavity itself, which could progress rapidly and even prove fatal.

'OK, Maddy, if you could just gently squeeze here' – I

passed her the portion of intestines in front of the mass – 'and then here' – I handed her a similar portion behind the mass – 'and now get comfortable!'

Both nurses chuckled.

To prevent seepage and contamination, the entry and exit points either side of the foreign body are temporarily occluded. (The gentle pressure applied between the soft index and middle finger of a human's hand is often considered the safest and most effective way to achieve this, rather than the unforgiving clamps of a metal surgical instrument. That is, as long as the volunteer's hand doesn't cramp up, or suddenly lose its grip.)

'Just be as quick as you can!' Maddy replied.

I stabbed my scalpel blade through a front portion of the bulging intestinal tissue, with the aim of pulling the offending item forwards. As I did, the walls of the intestine peeled away from each other, and a neon orange structure came into view, coated with greenish-brown intestinal contents.

'What the flippin' heck is that?' I asked Maddy, who was equally engrossed as we edged closer to revealing the big moment of truth.

I continued my incision and with a pair of forceps, I took hold of the orange tip but the teeth of my forceps cut through the soft foamy texture. I released the grip, realigned and repeated my grasp to gain a better purchase. I gently started to tease and edge the orange elongated cylinder along, through the hole I had created in the intestinal wall, then 'pop', the tension eased and in the grasped teeth of my forceps I had pulled a bright orange foam cylinder from Rocky's intestines.

'Not . . . a . . . clue,' Maddy replied.

With the pressure relieved, the loop of stretched intestine

recoiled and as a chameleon might change colour, it slowly converted from a deep maroon back to a calmer more normal-looking reddish pink, a good sign that the portion of gut was healthy enough to recover and shouldn't need cutting out.

I sutured the intestines, then, once Maddy had released her grip, squeezed some intestinal contents along the 'tube' to check for any leakage. Confident that things were as they should be, I flushed the abdomen, closed the muscle layer, the subcutaneous fat and eventually I closed Rocky's skin.

Once the operation was complete, and Rocky had been moved through to recovery, the excitement made me want to find out more about my newly discovered treasure. I ran the orange item under the tap – a foam cylinder, about two inches in length.

I called Emily with the good news that we *did* find something and that the surgery had all gone well. I described what we had found, then I ran through the aftercare, the monitoring and the importance of getting Rocky eating again. I talked through the medication he would come home on but then suddenly, 'Oh my God!' Emily interrupted the telephone conversation. 'I know exactly what *that* is!'

A couple of days previously, she had spotted her son playing what seemed like a fairly harmless game at the top of the staircase. He was firing the enticingly bright, foamy orange bullets down the hallway from his toy gun – which Rocky then 'hunted' down, one after the other, as the bullets (which were probably in a cat's mind about the size and texture of a small mouse) came flying along the carpet at a speed that Rocky could scramble after, pounce on and then all of a sudden 'gulp'. Rocky had decided to finish off his prey once and for all.

She assured me from then on they would be far more conscious of having anything around the house that might tempt Rocky's already pretty sharp hunting instincts, and then joked that the final invoice for Rocky's surgery made that Nerf gun the most expensive toy she had ever bought her son!

As I hung up the telephone and sat in the vet's office to pause for a moment, I can remember feeling so alive. I had completed surgery for the first time without the assistance of another vet. Rocky had come through. We'd solved the mystery. And I had learnt some of the subtleties of feline medicine and surgery. I was being requested by name by Ms Jeffries and had just removed an otherwise life-threatening obstruction from a cat's intestinal system. I was starting to gain some confidence, feeling like things were finally falling into place a little bit. For the first time, I felt like a *real* vet.

'James? JAMES?'

I heard Maddy call from the operating theatre. I looked over my shoulder and could see the two nurses huddled together by the operating table. They had their backs to me and were looking down at the table. Maybe Rocky had suddenly crashed in recovery? Did we need to start CPR? Where was the crash box if we needed it? How much adrenaline should I draw up? All the questions pinged through my mind. My brief bubble of confidence burst immediately as I ran from the vet's office, across the prep room, and over to assist Maddy with whatever disaster I was about to face.

I rushed into the operating theatre. Maddy, still with her back to me, suddenly turned around. The other nurse that had been assisting was cradling Maddy's right arm, helping her to keep her hand raised in the air. Maddy looked to be on the brink of fainting. And then I saw, clenched in her right hand, a blood-soaked swab leaching a trail of red liquid that streaked down the skin of her bare arm, exposed from the short-sleeved scrub top she had worn for the surgery.

'I just went to clear up the instruments . . . and . . . you . . . you'd left the scalpel on the tray.'

'What?' I replied. The guilt and fear that this was my fault suddenly shot through my body.

Maddy took a sharp inhale of breath through her clenched teeth, and flung her head back in pain. 'I've just . . . just cut the tip of my finger off. We . . . we need to go to hospital!'

'What? Oh my God, oh my God! Your finger?' I replied, leaping forwards to help steady Maddy, keep her upright and work out what to do. I darted my gaze around the theatre room floor to see if I could locate the accidentally amputated fingertip when suddenly Maddy snorted.

'Of course I haven't chopped my finger off, you bloomin' doughnut!'

Unable to hold character any longer, the two nurses began to laugh uncontrollably. Maddy threw the bloody swab at me. I realised then it was the same swab I had used through Rocky's surgery. They creased in laughter as I had fallen hook, line and sinker for their prank.

'But next time, take your sharps off the instrument tray when you've finished surgery!'

And with that, yet another lesson learnt.

CHAPTER 6

Rebel

For some time, I had been quite accustomed to living every day in crisis mode – it had become my 'norm'. Not just through the work-related anxieties that come with being a new grad vet either. For years, my life had been held suspended in a perpetual state of fight or flight from the anxiety that someone might find out who I 'really' was. That someone might unmask my truth and reveal my huge secret to the world. I was in my mid twenties, and my silence around my sexuality had started to speak volumes.

I didn't grow up in a homophobic household but I did grow up in a time when homophobia wasn't challenged by society. I was born in the 1980s, the peak Aids crisis; years filled with misinformation and bigotry; a time when fear and hatred towards homosexuality were rife. The only access to current affairs was through the television or the sensational-ist newspapers at the time, who regularly emblazoned their headlines with anti-LGBTQ+ fearmongering phrases such as 'terror', 'doom' and 'gay virus plague'. Gay marriage was illegal. Gay adoption was illegal. Section 28 prevented any discussion around homosexuality within schools. What did being gay even mean? And what would my future look like if I were to come out as gay? I knew I hadn't chosen to feel this way, it was just *in me*. But seeing these newspaper head-lines on our kitchen table, in our home, left unchallenged by society and with no internet or social media to offer any kind of counterview – it made my young mind realise the only choice I had was whether to confess to anyone that I felt this way or to keep it all to myself. And what would happen if I did tell anyone? Would I end up with 'the plague'? Would the life I loved with my animals and my family be 'doomed' for ever? Growing up, I didn't know a single gay person. I had no one to look up to. And so, when I began to question my sexuality – as a younger person often does – it's perhaps no surprise that I couldn't even say or hear the word 'gay' without setting off panic alarms in my mind.

I kept quiet for as long as I could. 'Coming out' was the single most daunting prospect I could have ever imagined. Eventually, in my early twenties, I tentatively gave it a go, but my first attempt was a complete, unmitigated disaster. I panicked, quickly brushed the whole thing under the carpet and ran straight back in the closet, for a long time too scared to ever try again. This 'gay shame' festered within me like a silent cancer. It ate away at my happiness, pushing me deeper and deeper into an unhealthy headspace until one evening alone in my flat in Jersey, having bottled everything up for far too long, I spiralled further than I ever had before. I found myself standing in front of my bedroom mirror at two in the morning, wearing nothing but my boxer shorts, with uncontrollable tears streaming out of my eyes. Naked, vulnerable and feeling completely alone, I put my head in my hands and cried and cried and cried. There was no lower I could go without devastating consequences. I know now that I had reached rock bottom.

For years I had hidden my struggles from everybody. I had shut myself off from friends and family; I had subconciously 'run away' to Jersey. On some level I think life took me that low to make me realise that mine was not a life I wanted to continue living. I knew I didn't want to die, but I also knew I didn't want to keep living the life that I was. Something had to change. I looked at my own reflection, stared into my own eyes – a poignant turning point in my life. I had a choice to make: keep running away or learn how to hold my head up high and find some pride in who I was. I had loved my time on Jersey, but despite feeling so much gratitude to the practice that raised me as a new graduate vet, I recognised that it was time for me to leave the isolation of island life, and return to the mainland. It was time to face up and start building a future of my own.

So, I did. I moved back to the UK and took a veterinary job in a practice that treated both horses and companion pet species. Of course, eventually the rumours caught up with me. I was outed at the practice I worked at and so I decided this time to own it. I came out for a second time. It wasn't any easier, it wasn't really even on my own terms, but by then I had witnessed several friends who had 'come out' and I had watched as their lives flourished. I began to covet their openness, I wanted to feel that same level of freedom and learn to live happily in my own skin. But also, by my second attempt I too felt more ready, because by then I had met Mark. We kept our relationship a secret at first, but he had already transformed my life for the better in ways I could never have imagined. Even though our relationship was only in its very early days, I knew in my heart I was already willing to sacrifice everything for him and so began a whole new chapter of my life.

'She's just round here. We've called her Rebel!'

I followed the young woman along the pebbled driveway, in front of their humongous Georgian mansion house, through the walled garden and eventually to the block of beautifully presented, tumbled-red-brick stables.

Chloe, still only in her mid to late twenties, was the daughter of the millionaire who owned the property and was herself an exceptionally talented professional horse rider and trainer. She was dressed in pale beige jodhpurs and a gilet jacket with the name of a well-known brand of horse feed stamped across the back, below which her surname had been embroidered. She was sponsored, knowledgeable and on track for greatness.

'I haven't got a clue what's happened,' Chloe said. 'I don't know whether she's put her head into something or she's been bitten, but I've never seen a reaction like it!' she continued, as I followed in her steps towards the stable door.

A few paces behind me, an eager third-year veterinary student called Rosie was listening in to the history as we began to gather our evidence for the clinical investigation. She had been shadowing me for a few weeks. It is a standard part of the course that all vet students have to complete a specific amount of time 'seeing practice', to help put the theoretical knowledge into a practical reality and learn some of the nuances around the art of veterinary science. As we approached the stable block, the young woman stopped outside a small room. I followed her in, thinking it perhaps led us to the next wing of their great estate. Rosie also dutifully followed suit.

I took in the familiar pine-wood-infused 'horsey' smell of the leather polish from the six shining saddles suspended from the wall, their accompanying bridles on hooks and a cabinet of medicines and supplements alongside them spanning the width of the room. A small but comfortable sofa I imagined to be the perfect place to pitch up for a mid-morning cuppa had already been claimed by an aged, content, curled-up German wirehaired pointer. 'Ooops, sorry,' Chloe said as she turned around, not expecting to see that both Rosie and myself had blindly followed her into the cramped space. In hindsight, it was only the size of a small garden shed – made even more awkward with the three of us crammed in there like sardines.

'I've just come in here to grab this,' she explained and reached across me to lift a sturdy-looking riding hat, complete with the same branding stamped across her gilet jacket.

I turned around and shuffled into Rosie, mouthing, 'Out! OUT!' like two wayward schoolkids that had stepped out of bounds.

We left the tack room and continued our walk towards the stable. 'I wouldn't normally wear this,' Chloe said as she lifted the riding hat to her head and buckled the strap beneath her chin, 'but she's a bit mardy even at the best of times, hence why she's called "Rebel"!'

As we approached the stable door, it was obvious the horse was flighty. She was pacing around the stable, round and round, then changing direction, light on her feet and whinnying.

'She's still a youngster,' Chloe said, as she began to heave and wiggle the heavy metal bolt of the stable door. 'I've only had her a few weeks, but she's thrown me off four times already,' she continued with a playful yet determined smirk. Most people would perhaps find that a terrifying warning sign, but for Chloe it showed the horse had drive. And a strong drive could be harnessed into huge potential.

The bolt slid along its metal casing with a loud clunk. Chloe used the toe of her wellington boot to flip a metal latch at the bottom of the stable door and manoeuvred her body quietly and elegantly through the small gap, then closed it behind her. Then she reached her arm over the door and locked herself in.

The young mare began to spin on the spot, aware of our presence, the whites of her eyes glaring and her nostrils widening in response to the unfamiliarity of what was happening. Chloe spoke in a hushed voice, an attempt to reassure the apprehensive animal. But as she crept closer, the slender chestnut mare continued to hop about on all four hooves, agitated, irritable and confused. As the horse continued to spin, Chloe quietly stepped forwards with a lead rope, but as she did so, the mare reared her front two feet off the ground in a slow but meaningfully threatening way.

Chloe's voice changed from her soft, calm demeanour as she grumbled a loud, strict 'NO!' towards the skittish mare. The transition from the fiery, high-energy life of a youngster to the more conditioned life of a seasoned eventer takes a lot of time and patience. I'd never heard Chloe shout at one of her horses before, but she was experienced, and was perhaps communicating in a way the young horse would be more accustomed to, having come straight from one of the more 'heavy-handed' dealers on the equine circuit.

It seemed to work, as Chloe continued to edge towards the mare, and despite the horse lifting its head to almost twice her height, she managed to clip the lead rope onto the head collar. Their relationship was still in its infancy. The last thing Chloe needed was the necessity of a vet visit to disrupt the small steps of progress she had made. But even from the stable door, I could see the horse was in desperate need of my veterinary attention.

'OK, she should be all right now if you want to come in,' Chloe called over to us as we hovered outside.

Not really, I thought to myself. Not one single ounce of me wanted to step inside the stable with the wild beast, but of course, the professional cap went on, I slid the bolt open and answered her with a confident, 'Sure.'

I stepped into the stable and took a couple of paces towards the horse. The autumnal midday light offered only the slightest assistance as I strained my eyes to assess the animal standing a few feet away. Rosie, too, was peering from over the stable door. The skin around the horse's eyes had swollen to such an extent that her eyelids were almost completely closed. Large, raised, doughnut-shaped wheals had popped up all down her neck, along her belly, over her hind quarters and almost down all four legs. And in between the larger areas of swelling, the rest of her skin had inflamed into hundreds of small, raised, itchy lumps, as though her skin had been stretched over some bubble wrap. The reaction had developed extremely quickly, in the previous hour or so. The horse had become immediately restless, refused food and was dancing on the spot – unable to comprehend why her skin felt so prickly. An allergic reaction, a severe allergic reaction, to an unknown trigger. Also known as a hives reaction – or urticaria. Of course, in a perfect world it would be helpful to somehow isolate the allergen (an insect bite or sting, a new shampoo or even a food allergy, for example) and avoid it in the future, but frustratingly the underlying cause is often never found and the focus, instead, moves to the more pressing urgency of getting the allergic reaction under control.

'She'd benefit from a steroid injection,' I said to Chloe, as I bent over, still standing a good seven or eight feet away, trying to peer a glance at the horse's underbelly. 'Ideally I'd like to get her heart rate, perhaps even check her gums to see their colour?'

I looked at Chloe. She didn't appear hugely hopeful.

'I'd also really like to try and get her temperature.' Chloe's eyes widened as if to say, 'Are you mad?' I wasn't particularly enamoured with the idea of casually waltzing up behind the panic-stricken animal and sticking a thermometer up its bum either, so reading Chloe's reaction, I continued, 'But I'm not sure we'll manage that, looking at how worked up she is. I'll see if she'll let me take her heart rate.' I pulled the stethoscope from around my neck and positioned the soft silicone buds in both of my ears. As I crept closer, though, the horse started sidestepping away. With my left hand I very slowly reached forwards to see if she would let me stroke down her neck. But as soon as my skin touched hers, her panic heightened further, the same knee-jerk reaction you might expect when you accidentally give a friend a static electric shock when you've just pulled a woollen jumper over your head. Except for the horse, her whole body was electric and sensitised, charged with an intense itchiness that was causing her skin to crawl. She leapt away from me and, using her full strength, she barged past and completed an entire loop of the stable, taking Chloe, who was still grumbling her strict commands into the horse's ear, with her.

'This might not be so easy,' I said out loud as I pulled the stethoscope from my ears and retired to the far corner of the stable again.

If I couldn't take her heart rate, couldn't get near her to check the colour of her gums, and couldn't get her temperature, how on earth would I get an injection into her?

'She's pretty good with needles,' Chloe replied, reading the situation and unpicking the perplexed grimace across my face. 'Honestly, she was fine for her vaccinations a couple of weeks ago. If that helps?' she said, almost apologetically.

All I needed to do was get an injection of corticosteroid into the horse to appease the reaction. I knew that within moments her skin would feel soothed and the swellings would start to subside. But how?

There were three options. Firstly, sedation. Chemical restraint is sometimes the only safe way to approach certain patients, but sedation *still* requires an injection of some kind. Secondly, do nothing. Hives reactions are rarely fatal and may even settle on their own accord as long as the allergen is taken away. But the poor horse looked like a pufferfish that had been stung by a million bumble bees. Not for one second did I expect Chloe would be comfortable with a hands-off approach. The clinical risks weren't hugely alarming, but it was incredibly distressing to see her horse like that. The third option would be to just try. Trust Chloe's handling skills and go for it.

Of course, Chloe was most game for the latter. Through

her otherwise incredibly successful career with horses, by the age of twenty-seven she had already broken three bones, had fifteen stitches across and down her left cheek, been taken to hospital in an air ambulance twice and spent six months in a neck brace. I wasn't sure whether that made her terrible at her job or a fearless master of her craft. But as my grandmother, a skilled horsewoman in her own youth, had said to me on many occasions at the riding school as a child, 'You'll never make a good rider until you've fallen off a few times.' I concluded that this proved that Chloe was exceptionally gifted with horses. And I should trust her.

So I went back to the car to draw up the calculated volume of clear, medicinal liquid into a syringe. I changed the needle, then dowsed a ball of cotton wool with some surgical spirit and returned to the stable block. The short space of time allowed me to mentally prepare myself for the imminent battle between me, horse and the safe administration of said intravenous corticosteroid injection.

'Rosie, I think it's probably best if you stay outside, if that's OK?' There is a legal responsibility on vets that basically says if anything happened to Rosie or Chloe, it would very likely be my head on the chopping block.

I stepped back inside the stable and followed Chloe's footsteps up to the front end of the mare. The two of us tried to stay on the same side of the horse so neither of us could get squished against a wall if she panicked. With my left hand I managed to stroke the ball of wet cotton wool along the jugular groove of the horse's neck, and then placed it in my pocket. The liquid quickly seeped through the thin cotton lining of my trousers and I felt the ice-cold surgical spirit make contact with my own skin. Then, using my left thumb,

I occluded the vein, which caused the sunken groove to rapidly swell to roughly the diameter of a hosepipe, running all the way from my thumb up to the horse's head.

'OK, girl, you're OK,' I said, as I focused my mind. She had responded well up to this point. I took the cap off the needle with my teeth (a terrible habit really but unfortunately, not being an octopus, and with only two hands available, it was a case of 'needs must'). Then I realigned my aim and, with the horse still hopping up and down on the spot, plunged the needle deep into her jugular vein. True to Chloe's word, the horse didn't seem to flinch at the needle itself, but she did still seem agitated at the general presence of everyone around her. Coupled with the fact her skin must have felt like she had a million ants scuttling all over her.

She took two steps forwards. We both moved with her – and I managed to keep the needle in position. Then I began to withdraw on the syringe plunger. Thick venous red blood entered the syringe, swirling and mixing with the clear corticosteroid medicine like a 1970s lava lamp. The presence of the blood proved to me the needle had remained within the central lumen of the vessel and was therefore correctly and safely positioned to administer the medication. I depressed the syringe plunger and the steroid injection flowed into her bloodstream.

'Well, that went better than I thought,' I said as I withdrew the needle and pressed my thumb against the puncture site. Chloe looked equally relieved.

I replaced the cap and disconnected the empty syringe from the needle, then turned to leave the stable. But as I did so, the mare's patience had worn thin. And suddenly I felt the huge gluteal muscles of the horse's rear end swing round and knock into my side. Like an enormous pendulum, her entire body swept from left to right across the width of the stable, taking me out in its path. I managed to stay standing but had been trapped between the stable wall and the horse's powerful hindquarters.

Chloe resumed her low grumbly teacher voice, accompanied with various growls and groans and repeatedly offered a 'Wooooah, girl!' and 'Nooooo!', but with a much lesser effect. I looked over my shoulder at the exact same time the chestnut mare reared her front feet off the ground, then as her front feet fell back down to the wood shavings, her rear end bunny hopped skywards into a bucking motion, only a couple of feet away from my head, as she kicked her back legs out behind her. One of her hind hooves made contact with the wooden panelled wall of the stable. Thankfully, the panels held their strength despite the impact under such force. But the loud bang spooked the horse even more. Like a 'bucking bronco' ride at a carnival, she reared and then bucked, and then reared again, moving round on the spot like the dials of a clock, with Chloe at her head end, and me trapped near the rear.

'THE DOOR!' I called to Rosie, who thankfully acted with lightning speed.

Suddenly, as Chloe had one hand on the lead rope and placed her other against the pectoral muscle of the mare, I felt the wind taken from me. The kick came flying at me with such an incredible velocity. All I can remember is feeling the brush of the hoof as it made contact. I looked down at the fleece I was wearing and almost in a slow motion *Matrix*-style stunt move, my whole body seemed to fold in half at the hips as I flew backwards.

The horse's metal shoe had only managed to make a relatively narrow point of impact across my sternum. A full-contact, full-impact kick and I would have been squished like a fly. Instead, I fell backwards towards the door and heard another 'bang' as the momentum of the hoof (which continued along the same trajectory path I was falling) smashed into the wooden stable door. Thankfully, with Rosie the student's lightning response to unbolt the door, the impact of the hoof caused the stable door to fly wide open and through it I came tumbling outside, landing in a heap on the cobbled ground. A bruised arse and a pretty significant graze across the chest I could cope with. But I do still wonder, if that door had remained bolted shut, and Rosie the vet student hadn't been there, how different the outcome might have been.

Chloe managed to release the lead rope and soon followed me out of the stable.

'Shit, I'm so sorry!' she said.

'Occupational hazard!' I joked back, dusting myself off and trying to override the burning sensation from the grazes on both of my palms. I have no shame in admitting I was pretty shaken up. It was a real wake-up call. Sitting in a heap on the cobbled stones in a pool of yellow-brown horse piss that had leached from the stable bedding, I looked at Chloe and thought how stupid of me not to carry my own hard hat in the car. It is so easy as 'the vet' to focus solely on the task in hand and kind of forget that actually, sometimes, it's an incredibly dangerous job. One study even cited equine veterinary practice as the most dangerous civilian occupation, ahead even of working in the fire or prison service. Lesson learnt (ish).

I stood up, still slightly trembling as the sudden surge of adrenaline gently dissipated, wiped myself off and headed back to the car with Rosie.

As we drove to our next call and discussed the various differentials around what may have triggered the hives reaction and dissected every second of the 'kick', I spent most of the journey thanking Rosie for her quick thinking. As with most times when someone falls flat on their arse, we also had a good laugh at my expense. It's definitely not one to forget: the horse that kicked the vet out of its stable! 'Do you have horses?' I asked Rosie, knowing she was considering entering equine practice after graduating. The answer was no, but she had grown up around them. She returned the question. Then she asked if I had any pets.

It struck me at the time as such an obvious question, and one that I really ought to have a better answer to. Ever since leaving home, going to uni, taking the first job in the Channel Islands and then moving back to the mainland, I guess it seemed quite obvious that my lifestyle didn't quite suit having a pet. But when Rosie asked me that day, I remember feeling disappointed that my answer was 'no'.

For a while, I had been feeling like I was hankering for something. Like something was missing. Being a vet is so wonderful in so many ways, but as an animal lover, it was quite a bitter pill: to train for so long, then spend all day, every day, surrounded by sick, ill, injured or frightened animals. I make them better, but once they have returned to health, I don't get to follow my patients home and see them running on the beach, curled up by the fire, enjoying their evening treat or achieving great things on an agility course. Those precious moments are shared between a pet owner and their pet, the 'human–animal bond'. As a vet, I was too busy already seeing the next wave of sick, injured or frightened animals. And having grown up surrounded by lots of animals, I realised that was what I was missing. I needed my own dog. A dog to love. A dog to give love in return. I needed to get back to the simple enjoyment of spending time in the company of a *healthy* animal.

'I don't have a pet, no,' I replied to Rosie, 'but I'd love to get a dog.'

'What breed?' she asked.

'Hmm, my guilty pleasure would be a tiny chihuahua.' We both laughed. 'But in all honesty, I think if I could choose any breed, it would have to be a Labrador.' I've always loved Labradors. Their kind nature, their docile temperament and their lovely square heads and squidgy jowls. They are, in my mind, the perfect 'all-round' dog.

'I love Labs too,' Rosie shrieked. 'My sister's Lab has just had a litter.'

I took a punt. 'Are any still available?' I asked, half in jest and half in hope.

'No, sadly they all went to their new homes this weekend,' Rosie said. 'Well, actually, there is one puppy left but he's got a bit of a sad story, one of the male pups.'

'What happened?' I asked.

'One of her other Labs, who can be a bit funny with other dogs, took him from the litter, and just, sort of, attacked him when he was only six weeks old.'

I briefly took my eyes off the road and looked at her with the same expression that everyone makes when they hear about a baby animal falling on hard times – that sort of frowning, sad clown face.

'I know,' she said. 'Apparently she just picked him up in her mouth and shook him.'

'WHAT?!' I shouted, outraged.

'Yeah, he fell against the radiator and fractured his jaw, I think. Lost an eye too. I'm not sure what she's thinking of doing with him. Whether to keep him or not, but I think he's doing OK now. I'll see if I've got a photo.'

When we parked, Rosie reached into her rucksack and pulled out a flip phone, then turned the screen to show me.

'Oh . . . my . . . GOD!' I replied.

I had expected to be shown a rather terrifying, bloody image of a six-week-old puppy with an eye hanging out and a misaligned jaw. It is part of the territory, vet to vet, that gruesome photos become the norm – a kind of 'clinical knowledge sharing' in pictorial form. A horrific wound or a broken leg or a vast quantity of haemorrhagic diarrhoea shown on a screen by a colleague who'd then very casually ask, 'What would you do with this?' But when I looked at Rosie's screen, there was no blood. No dangling eyeball. No messy trauma case to comment on. Just a grainy image of the most adorable, innocent-looking, fluffy yellow Labrador puppy – sitting and peering out from an alcove in a kitchen, with his head gently tilted to one side and his one remaining teddy-bear brown eye looking up at the camera with a hopeful glint and a cheeky sparkle.

'Wow,' I said, with a chuckle at how ridiculously adorable the puppy seemed.

After that I bombarded her with questions, but sadly, it being her sister's litter of puppies, Rosie eventually had to stop me. 'Honestly, I don't know that much!' she insisted. 'The last I heard a vet nurse had shown some interest but I don't know how far they got.'

My heart sank. What was happening? I'd never met this puppy. I didn't even know he existed until a few minutes ago. Yet when I heard someone else might be taking him on, I was devastated. I'd always hoped a dog would just kind of come into my life, and it felt like this puppy could be the one. In fact, in my mind in that moment, he *was* the one.

As we finished our last call of the day, I gave Rosie my email address. And hoped.

Then a few days later, an email arrived:

James and Mark,

I understand from my sister that you may be interested in my one-eyed Lab pup, nine-week-old male Star (Starbright Edwards). He is an absolute sweetie with a lovely temperament, it's just a shame that the accident happened and now he only has one eye and as a consequence will grow with a deformed head. Mentally and physically, though, he seems to be very well and has recovered remarkably quickly. I have tried to convince my mum but she is not in the right place to have him and as my pack is already full I can't keep him (sadly).

I have attached a link to our page of photos. I don't have any up-to-date ones but there is also a picture of Mum (Willow) and Dad (Max). Both beautiful working-type Labs. Both have current eye certificates and have brilliant hip/elbow scores. Dad was also screened for CNM (by parentage, I think). Star is Kennel Club registered and has been wormed and will have been fully vaccinated.

I need to meet you and of course you will need to see him. He will be £250 (they were £550 full price).

Please understand that I am keen to find him the perfect home (which I am sure you will be) and that I want to stay in touch with him over the next few months to see that he makes a full recovery, though I don't anticipate that there will be any problems.

Hope you are still interested,

Charlotte

I read it over and over, opening each of the photos time and time again. I showed Mark, and he was equally besotted. We exchanged further emails. Then, that weekend, we made a plan to meet.

As we arrived, we met the family and were invited through to the kitchen where we first met Mum: a beautiful golden Labrador. She immediately picked up her favourite toy and carried it across the kitchen in her mouth, doing the happy Labrador 'wiggle-bottom' dance with her hips.

Following a few paces behind came her last remaining puppy. I peered round hoping to catch a glimpse of the gentle-looking fluffball of a pup we had seen in the photo, but he was running so fast behind Mum, under the kitchen table, round the chair legs, into the next room then back again, that I only caught a glimpse. As he came back round the corner, I saw him for the very first time. Cute, yes, but not *quite* like the angelic puppy in the photo. Through all the anticipation, we had built quite a strong picture in our mind of who we were there to see. We were expecting to meet the small, docile Andrex puppy with the button nose and the winking eye. Just like in the photo we had grown obsessed with. He looked cuddly and calm. But of course, in the photo, he was only six weeks old.

Instead, we were greeted by a gangly eleven-week-old ball of restless energy with a scrunched-up face, who hated being held still and just wanted to play. He wanted to wrestle. He wanted to chomp on things and bark at things and run at things. He had one eye open and from the socket of the missing eye streamed a dark brown tearstain that cascaded from the inside corner of his eyelid and down his face. He looked like a teenager that had got into a fight and was ready and raring for round two. He quickly grew bored of our staring and used all his might to pull the foam stuffing out of his crocodile-shaped soft toy.

'He's changed a lot, hasn't he?' I said tentatively to Charlotte.

'He certainly has! You can see the accident doesn't seem to have held him back, though, he's full of beans!'

She wasn't wrong!

'But he does really need to get into a new home now and start his proper training.'

Absolutely he did! It was agreed that if we would like him, Charlotte would be willing to let us take him. It's a funny thing when you go to meet a puppy. Everyone says to think with your head and not your heart. I looked at the defenceless, slightly feral-looking creature, as he chewed at my sock and nipped at my big toe and thought, *am I definitely sure about this?* I will confess, there was a small seed of doubt in my mind. He was a much livelier character than I'd imagined. He'd also be the first dog of my own and Mark's first dog ever and, with his scrunched-up little face and unknown level of possible long-term brain damage from the accident, was he perhaps too much for us to take on as first-time dog dads? Would he be too much of a handful for us to cope with?

'What do you think you would call him?' Charlotte asked.

'Well . . . we think he'd suit Oliver,' Mark replied.

'Oliver,' I said quietly, as I knelt down to pick him up. In my mind, it was going to be the 'Simba' moment, like in *The Lion King*: I would raise my son up and bless him into our family. But as I lifted Oliver, he contorted his neck in every direction, like the child from *The Exorcist*, mouthing my hands with his little crocodile teeth.

'Ooh, ow!' I put him back on the ground. And he continued to nip at my toes.

'What do you think?' I said to Mark, who by now looked like a child whose wildest dreams had just come true.

'I love him,' he replied instantly. 'He's perfect!'

Perfect? I smiled. And laughed. The one thing about Mark is that he has an innate ability to only ever see the positive in *any* situation. I agreed, though. I loved him too. I loved his rebellious streak and was up for the challenge. So, with a great leap of faith, we handed over the money, signed the contract and changed his name on the microchip paperwork from 'Star' to 'Oliver'.

Moments before we had left, we'd taken Oliver into the garden with his mum for a toilet break. It was a good call, as not only did he squat down in exactly the same way his mother did and take a giant pee, moments later, with his nose to the ground, he circled the lawn and adopted the 'other' position as he curled out a stinky brown number. 'Better out than in!' Charlotte said, in an attempt to break the awkwardness around five human beings all staring at an eleven-week-old puppy take a dump on their lawn. And while it is absolutely true that 'what goes in, must come out', I think most of us would agree that 'what comes out should never really go back in'!

Unless, of course, you are Oliver.

As soon as he had finished his business, he spun on the spot and faster than anyone could react, immediately gobbled up what he had just produced.

'Ew,' I said. 'That was . . . speedy!'

Charlotte had started to notice this habit since he'd seen his mother eat the faeces of his litter mates. It's not unusual, especially for those puppies that have stayed with the mothers longer than most would normally. But it can be a tricky habit to break. And although not necessarily dangerous to a dog's health, it's always a bit revolting to watch.

Nevertheless, I climbed into the passenger seat, and we parcelled him onto my lap. As we drove off, I pulled his soft velvet ears through my fingers and watched as our new little puppy drifted off into a deep sleep. I smiled at Mark. Before long the motion and rocking of the ride home became too much for Oliver's little stomach to handle. After about ten minutes, he suddenly rose to his feet and began the classic swaying forwards then backwards, his stomach started contracting and then came the pumping, hiccupping noise that invariably predicts vomit is on the way.

'Oh no! I think he's going to be sick,' I said to Mark, who was by now driving along the main dual carriageway.

And then, sure enough, up came a large volume of foody vomit. But it wasn't just his dog food he brought up.

'What's that smell?' Mark asked.

'Oh no, open the window!' I shouted at Mark while I looked down at the pile of brown solid faecal-vomit on my lap.

'Bloody 'ell, that STINKS!' he replied, with his Midlands twang.

I could feel the liquid fraction of the vomit seep through my chino trousers. Oliver's face looked frail as his queasiness continued. Mark reached to the footwell and grabbed an old empty crisp packet. Then, as I held on to Oliver, he pushed his hand into the crisp packet the same way someone might use a 'poo bag' and grabbed a handful of the offending poo-vomit from the V-shaped gulley between my legs. With one hand on the steering wheel, Mark's other hand hovered in front of me at head height, his clenched fist in a crisp packet holding on to a handful of puppy vomit mixed with faeces, he shook it and shouted, 'Take it off me!'

I tried. I attempted to peel the crisp packet from his hand, but there just wasn't enough 'give' in the silver foil to pull it over his fist. He slightly loosened his grip on the vomit, and I continued to pull the crisp packet over his hand, then suddenly he let go. I felt the packet loosen. Between the force of me pulling and Mark withdrawing, we had essentially created a sling shot, which catapulted the mound of poo-vomit through the air until it slapped straight into the passenger side door handle.

'AAAAAGHHH!' I looked down at the mess around me.

Immediately I started gipping,* over and over.

The stench of dog vomit mixed with faeces is incomparable and I had no choice but to hang my head out of the window to stop myself from vomiting on the spot. Mark did the same on his side. Eventually he pulled off at the next exit and we both flung the car open and leapt out of the car.

---

* 'Gipping' is the Yorkshire, and therefore proper, word for 'retching'.

With Oliver in my arms, and a faeces-mixed-with-dog-vomit-smear down both of my trouser legs, across the majority of the dashboard of the car and all over the passenger door and seat, we stood on the side of the road and looked at each other. Not quite the romantic start we had hoped for or envisaged, but there was no going back. Oliver had firmly established himself as part of our family. For the two of us, he *was* our family. And despite the less from ideal journey home, from that moment onwards, we had made a commitment that we would love him. Warts 'n' all.

CHAPTER 7

Bob and Jill

Unlike most puppies, it wouldn't be that unheard of for our tiny one-eyed Oliver puppy to occasionally run head first into a misjudged chair leg, an 'invisible' lamp post, or on one occasion, our television screen, having spotted a fellow two-dimensional canine in the corner of his lounge.

We protected him as best we could, removed any obstacles, laid cushions in his path and wrapped towels around the sharp table legs – but the occasional clonk on the head, followed by a high-pitched puppy 'halp' became the symbolic sound that another lesson had been learnt in puppyhood and served as a reminder that he saw the world a little differently to most other dogs.

With time, his spatial awareness grew stronger and stronger and with each week that passed, his own intuition took over as he learnt to navigate the world at just a fractionally slower pace. There were a few mishaps, of course. Like the time he got his head stuck in the mouth of an empty plastic watering can. The vision from the kitchen window of a bright green watering can flailing wildly around the garden, having taken on a paranormal life of its own, stopped me in my tracks – until I spotted the big blob of golden fluff it was attached to!

His overall coordination, though, did always remain a little shy of what others might consider 'normal'. As he grew to a young teenager, we'd managed to teach him to 'give a paw' – but rather than a neat paw being offered into the palm of my hand, a huge walloping limb came flying out in front of him as he could never quite discern where my hand began and his paw ended. He would throw his entire front left leg in a wide arc out in front of him, in any general direction, in the understanding that at some point it meant getting a treat!

His depth perception, having only one eye, was something that proved a constant challenge to his day-to-day life. For the large part it never held him back. He used his paws to 'feel' in front of him. He'd dip his toe into the edge of a puddle to try to work out what it was. Or use his foot to tentatively 'tap' the ground in front of him – a cobbled street, for example, caused great confusion to him. Any sort of bridge, though, especially a bridge over moving water, was Oliver's arch nemesis. 'C'mon, Oliver, it's OK,' we would say, to try to reassure and entice him towards the foot of the bridge with treats. The closest we could reach would be to have one paw on the first step and then inevitably, at the very last minute, out of fear he would turn on the spot and run in the opposite direction. It became normal for one of us to heave a trembling Oliver up into our arms, no matter how muddy, carry him *over* the bridge in a firefighter's embrace and deposit him on the other side. On touchdown, he was straight away full of the joys of spring once more, leaping around and barking, congratulating us all on our successful completion of the most epic voyage to cross the most treacherous, dangerous river bridge. If there were a bottle of champagne to hand, he would have popped it there and then, and sprayed us all with foam at our heroic team achievement! Sadly, we never quite managed to convince him that it was *just* a bridge!

When it came to teatime, though, he was a typical Labrador through and through. His obsession with food meant he had an unfortunate habit of jumping up. As a little puppy, jumping up with his paws held out in front of him might sound endearing, but eventually having thirty-seven kilograms of adult Labrador jump up and wallop you in the nuts twice a day made feeding times an increasingly painful affair.

So, thanks to some additional training, instead of him jumping up *at* us, he learnt to jump up *in front* of us, on the spot, like a child doing star jumps in PE. Throughout his entire life, at even the slightest hint of food, his paws would lift, as though he was climbing onto a pogo stick, and he would bounce on the spot, with all four feet leaving the ground, until some food arrived in his bowl. And, having recognised that there were perhaps some developmental challenges to his overall mental capacity following his head injury as a puppy, we decided it was a fair compromise to settle on. The teatime 'Tigger bounce', as we called it, became one of his trademark moves.

With all of our family either in Yorkshire or the Midlands, it was quite normal for us to spend a lot of time travelling. Thankfully, Oliver quickly adapted to life on the road, having accompanied me daily from an early age on my horse calls. Having returned late on a Sunday evening from a long weekend up North, I lifted the car boot and released him from his crate. He ran straight to the back door. I let him in and decided the simplest way to keep him distracted while we emptied the luggage from the car was to fill his food bowl and let him tuck into an evening meal. I served. He bounced. He ate.

On one particular Sunday, that awful sinking 'Sunday blues' feeling had well and truly set in; the excitement of the weekend was over, just a distant memory, leaving behind a hangover, a bloated gut and a suitcase full of dirty laundry. But as Mark and I sulked our way back into the house, carrying the last few pieces of luggage from the car, it was clear that the weekend drama was only just beginning.

'What the . . .?' I walked through the kitchen door and dropped the rucksack from my shoulder in utter disbelief. Oliver, the same dog who refused to climb stairs or cross over a bridge, had from somewhere mustered the agility and bravado of a mountain goat – and was now standing *on top* of the kitchen table. Like a majestic bronze statue, he had his four feet placed wide apart, balanced perfectly on the tabletop, his nose snuffling through some tin foil. Aghast, I stood and watched him, strangely proud of his epic bravery. I called Mark to come and share in our boy's achievement – knowing full well he wouldn't believe me unless he witnessed it with his own eyes.

Tin foil though? Where's he found that? I asked myself. And then it dawned on me. We had stopped en route to see my godmother, who had kindly fuelled our onward journey with a homemade cake. I'd carefully placed it in the middle of the table, supposedly out of the reach of Oliver, but it seemed he had spotted his prize and confronted his fears

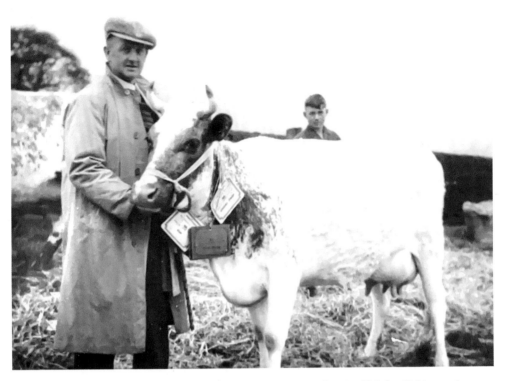

Tom Pickles, my great-grandfather. 'Best cow or heifer in calf' at the Hebden Bridge and Calder Valley Agricultural Show, 1958.

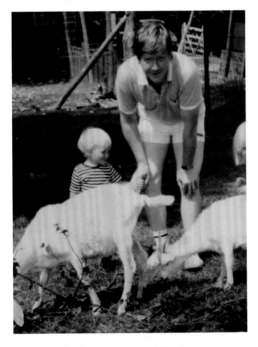

Dad introducing me as a toddler to a couple of friendly goats (perhaps where my obsession began?!) on a family holiday to Devon, 1986.

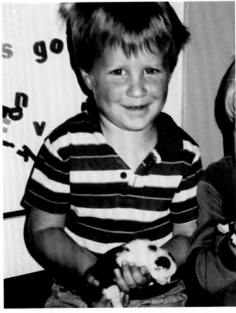

Huddersfield, June 1987. I loved visiting my godmother Melissa's house, also full of animals, here with their new kitten Panda. They also had a cockatiel called Tufty who lived to an incredible twenty-eight years old.

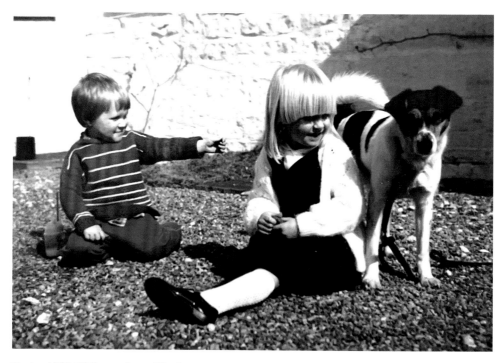

Easter 1986. With my sister, Nicola, on one of our many family holidays to Filey with our granny and grandpa's dog Shambles – named because she was an unknown mix of many different breeds.

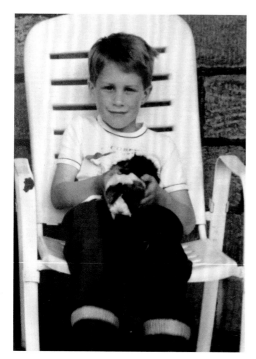

Huddersfield, 1991. Holding Scruffy the guinea pig, my first beloved pet that wasn't a goldfish!

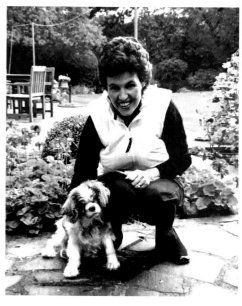

Huddersfield, 2003. Mum with our first dog, Smudge, a kind-natured King Charles Spaniel who must have been close to thirteen by the time the photo was taken. She arrived when I was seven and died when I was twenty – a huge part of my youth.

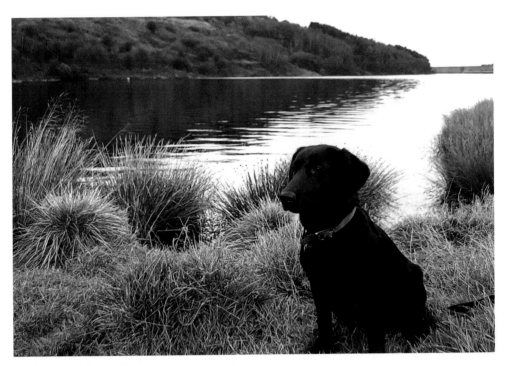

Scammonden Reservoir, West Yorkshire, 2004. After Smudge came Maisie. She was born on a farm in North Yorkshire and was a fantastic, energetic and loyal dog, brilliantly responsive and a great companion.

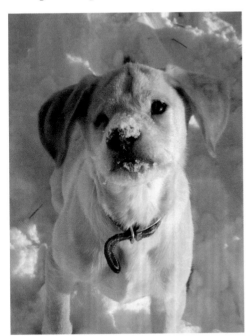

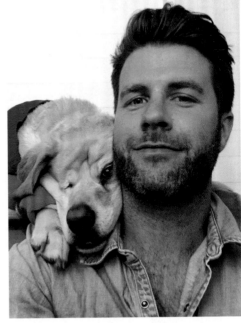

Hope Valley, Derbyshire, 2009. A twelve-week-old Oliver and his first experience of snow, snuffling his nose through it or trying to eat it!

Bristol, 2018. With Oliver as I practised my skills in the pottery shed, him offering me some moral support as he watched yet another handful of clay fly off the wheel!

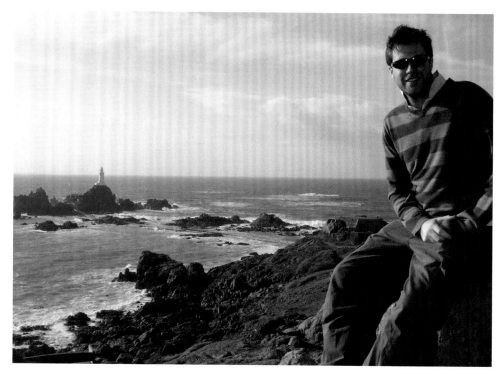

Le Corbière Lighthouse, Jersey, 2008. A stunning and favourite spot to sit and watch either the crashing tides or the panoramic stillness of a fiery sunset.

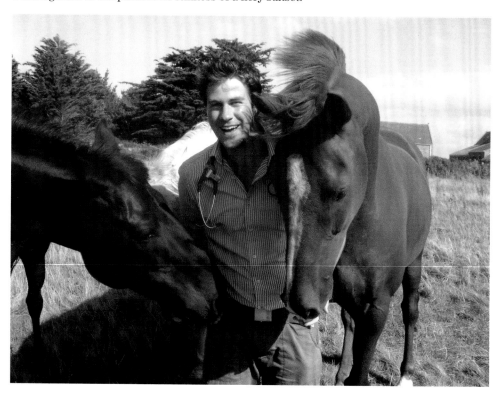

Horses in Jersey, 2008. With some of my first ever equine patients!

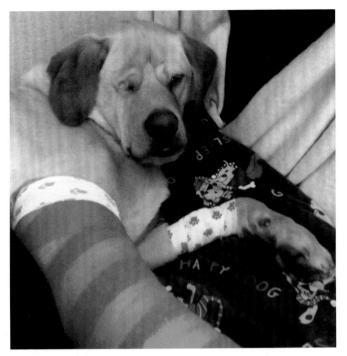

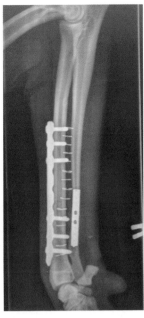

Bristol, 2010. A 'teenage' Oliver recovering from surgery after his car accident, snoozing through his pain relief medication and at the beginning of a slow eight-week recovery.

Bristol, 2010. A post-operative X-ray showing the orthopaedic metal work used to stabilise Oliver's fractured front leg.

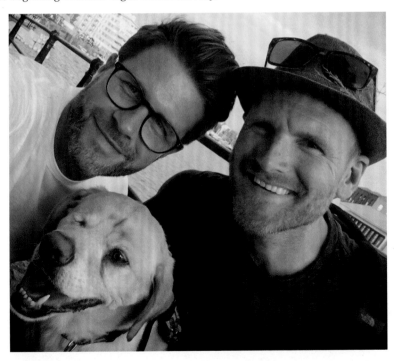

Bristol, 2017. Mark and I taking Oliver for a Sunday stroll around Bristol Harbourside, one of his favourite places as he got to meet so many adoring people!

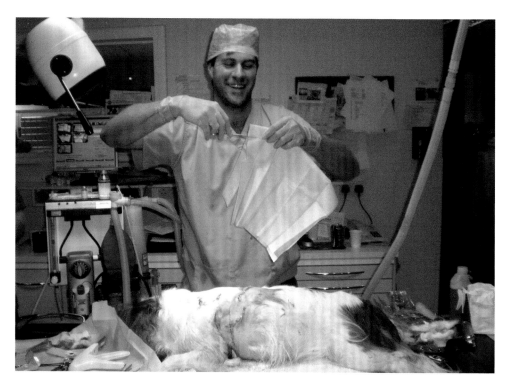

Jersey, 2007. Performing surgery as a new graduate vet – stitching up wounds from a dog that had charged through a fence, causing multiple skin lacerations.

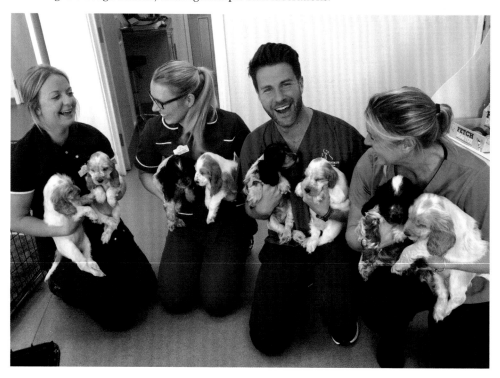

Bristol, 2017. A firm favourite among the veterinary team when a healthy litter of responsibly bred puppies arrive for their first vaccinations.

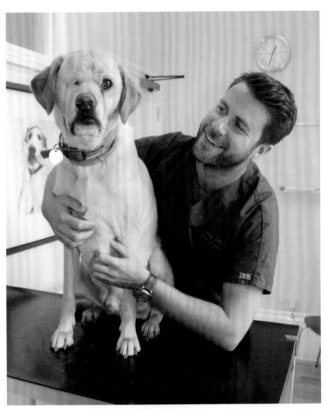

Left Bristol, 2015. In my consulting room at a lovely practice with a fantastic team. An added benefit was that I was allowed to bring Oliver to work with me!

Below North Yorkshire, 2018. Spring lambing time on a farm near Whitby.

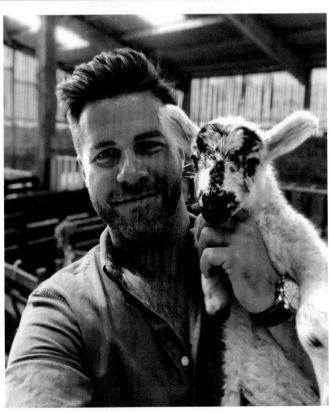

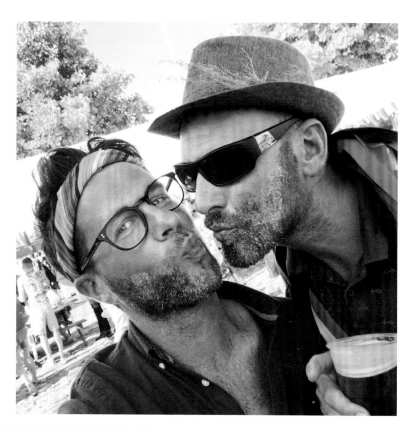

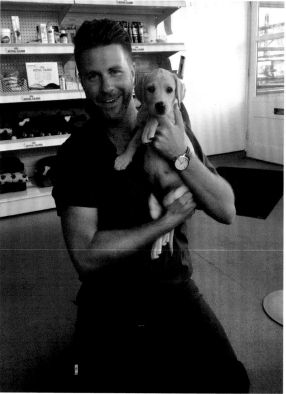

Above Bristol Pride, 2017. Mark and I together supporting our brilliant home city to celebrate love and inclusivity for all.

Left Bristol, 2017. Definitely a perk of the job, a Labrador puppy comes in for an early health check.

to sample a slice of chocolatey (and therefore *highly toxic*), sugary heaven.

In the land of veterinary medicine, having to phone your boss at 9.35 p.m. on a Sunday to let you into the practice because your *own* dog has eaten an *entire* chocolate cake, believe me, is quite a humbling experience! With Mark as my assistant, we arrived at the practice in the dead of night and after a quick injection into Oliver's scruff, soon found ourselves clearing up the various mounds of chocolatey vomit from the prep room floor. The only saving grace was that at least chocolate vomit is the one (and perhaps only) type of animal vomit that does actually smell quite pleasant.

Most animal mishaps or emergencies start with a phone call to the practice, swiftly followed by a rapid dash to the surgery. But then there are those pets in such urgent need of attention that an owner has no time (and often no thinking space) to call ahead and instead will just turn up.

For someone normally as impeccably dressed as Mrs Wainwright, I was surprised to greet her on the practice doorstep looking somewhat dishevelled. To put it bluntly, she looked like a drowned rat; dripping wet and with sprigs of duckweed still stuck in her hair, her fringe had plastered itself to her forehead and her spectacles were perched on the bridge of her nose at half-mast.

'Av just fell in mi pond!' she said, with her familiar Yorkshire twang. I'd always felt we had a strong bond thanks to our shared Yorkshire ancestry. Her ten-week-old shih-tzu poodle cross puppy, commonly known as a 'shih-poo' (or 'shittypoo' as she called her), looked equally sodden in her arms, but with a mischievous wag in her tail. Mrs Wainwright recalled how her puppy had sneakily followed her out into the garden. As she threw a handful of pelleted fish food into the water, she spotted the little floof ball at her feet peering into the deep. She spun around to avoid stepping on her new little companion, but lost her footing and instead toppled straight over the water's edge to join her koi carp. Worse, the puppy, who wasn't meant to be allowed anywhere near the pond, jumped straight in after her.

'Oh my God!' I replied. 'Are you OK?'

'Oh, I'm absolutely fine,' she said, 'just a bruised bloomin' ego! I'm pretty sure she's absolutely fine too.' She lifted the puppy in the air in front of her and looked her up and down. 'She *is* a little shittypoo, I tell yer . . . in more ways than one. The little scoundrel!' The puppy wagged its soggy wet tail ferociously in response to all this drama, flicking pond water over both of us.

'Actually, to be honest, I don't really know why I'm 'ere!' she said, looking around herself before cracking into a wide smile. 'I just didn't really know what else to do. I guess I just panicked and thought, I must get to the vet's!'

I offered a cursory, quick check of the puppy on the house – and, as predicted, all was absolutely fine. Mrs Wainwright stood soaked to the bone, the ten-week-old puppy did zoomies around my consulting room and all I could offer was a fresh dog towel from the kennel laundry and a calming cup o' tea. And, of course, a good giggle.

Giggles aside, there are other times when the situation is far more serious. When an owner will instead come rushing through the practice doors, clutching their pet in their arms and desperately calling out for help. It is in these moments the reception staff, a veterinary nurse or a fellow colleague will switch into 'triage' mode and the GP vet's surgery swiftly transforms itself into a fully functional A and E department. The adrenaline hits and the whole veterinary team diverts their focus to the pet that has been rushed in.

'Can we get some oxygen, please?' I called out to the veterinary nursing team, who had already begun the process of switching between their roles to receive the new emergency, a dog called Bob. One nurse stayed by the kennel side of the young tabby cat who was coming round from a routine cat spay, while the three others, currently on less pressing tasks, were able to drop everything and assist with the triage.

In my arms, a crossbreed rescue dog – a Jack Russell terrier crossed with a plethora of other breeds (a combination otherwise affectionately known in the trade as a 'Heinz 57'!). Sweet-natured Bob, a mix of white, caramel and black wiry fur and about twelve kilos of usually energetic and playful mischief, lay draped, unresponsive across my forearms as he drifted in and out of consciousness. He was unaware of his surroundings as he tremored with juddery, unpredictable muscle spasms that radiated across his entire body, as though someone was intermittently zapping him with a bolt of electricity from a remote-controlled button somewhere.

I lay his body down onto the mat of soft towelling on the table while the nurses hovered a mask over his muzzle so that with each breath, his red blood cells could saturate their haemoglobin with as much life-preserving oxygen as possible. Another nurse began to clip the fur from his left front leg and placed an intravenous cannula into his cephalic leg vein. I reached for a stethoscope – and listened over his heart and chest. Nothing abnormal, other than his heart rate that raced at one hundred and forty beats per minute. His eyes were fixed in a glazed forwards stare, as his body lay recumbent and tremoring. He could not follow my finger or the smell of a treat in front of his nose, but he could locate and respond to a whistle or a clap of the hands with a moderate move of his eyes – so not *entirely* unconscious. He also maintained control of his bladder and bowels and therefore overall was not the classic presentation for a seizure or 'fit', as a first impression might suggest.

I continued to check through his vital parameters and attempted to piece together in my mind what could be going on. 'I've got no idea,' I said under my breath to the nurse. 'He's not fitting, but he's definitely neurological.'

I took a thermometer and passed the metal tip into his back end. The reading beeped at 40.1 degrees centigrade. He was hot. And potentially going to get hotter and hotter if I didn't treat the muscle tremors promptly. The muscle tissue that connected his bony skeleton spontaneously contracted and relaxed with a chaotic rhythm that made his entire body spasm with tremors. The movement was involuntary, but it would still exert the same physiological effect on the body as a muscle undergoing exercise. Imagine running a marathon on a malfunctioning treadmill, out of control, and with no way of jumping off. His whole body – muscle, organs, heart, and eventually his brain – would get hotter and hotter, and eventually completely overheat with exhaustion. At which point his condition would rapidly become fatal. With each minute that passed, the risk increased that his temperature would continue to rise. His condition was a true emergency in every sense of the word.

'Let's get him on some fluids,' I said to the nursing team, who nodded in a coordinated and cooperative response.

With the nurse managing to restrain Bob's neck and keep it still, I drew enough blood from his jugular vein to fill two one-inch plastic tubes. The nurse gently agitated the blood tubes to prevent the precious dark red liquid from clotting. An in-house laboratory machine allowed us to check his organ function on a biochemistry reading, his electrolyte levels and his red and white blood cell haematology. As I continued my examination and calculated an appropriate drip rate of saline to begin flowing into Bob's circulatory system, my senior colleague Gemma walked through the prep room doors.

'Crikey, who's this we have here?' she asked, looking down at the wiry ball of tremoring terrier in between us.

Even though I had a few years under my belt, I can still remember feeling the huge amount of pressure I put on myself that I should be fully competent to tackle anything that walked through the door from day one. Of course, this was wholly unrealistic. Experience can only build with time, and through that process it's completely expected to draw upon insight from colleagues. But at the time, trying to come up with the differentials as to why Bob was tremoring on the table in front of me, something new that I had never seen before, took me straight back to feeling like a new grad vet once again. The constant rollercoaster of whether I was or wasn't a 'good enough vet'. Every day I felt like I needed the reassurance that I wasn't about to massively screw up while holding an animal's life in my hands. And with Bob, I was genuinely struggling to fit together any kind of reasoning for his cluster of urgently deteriorating symptoms.

'He was rushed in about ten minutes ago,' I said to Gemma. 'A six-year-old crossbreed, male, neutered, acute onset collapse and muscle tremors, hyperthermic. But he doesn't seem to have progressed into a full tonic-clonic seizure. He is still responsive but err, err, only ish, and I s'pose he's partly unconscious . . . but . . .'

There was something reassuring about rattling off the list of symptoms I'd uncovered – as though it somehow distracted my own mind from the fact I didn't have the foggiest clue in terms of a diagnosis. But the further down the list I rattled, the more confused I became.

I looked at Gemma. 'D'yer think it could be something toxic?' I took a punt, hoping if I offered at least one sensible solution, she might at least take pity and help me out.

Gemma knelt at the front end of the table and peered into the dog's fixed eyes. She used her thumb and forefinger to steady the upper and lower eyelids, then examined Bob's pupillary light reflex. 'Yeah, he looks toxic to me too,' she confirmed. 'If I were to hazard a guess, I'd say he's possibly eaten something.'

Gemma rose from her kneeled position and reached for the stethoscope. Looking down at the juddering dog in front of us, she paused and empathetically said, 'He's in a pretty bad way, isn't he?

'What do you think?' Gemma asked.

I rattled through a list of potential differentials in my mind as to why Bob might be tremoring. 'Maybe some mouldy food? A tremorgenic mycotoxin?'

She nodded. 'Definitely a possibility.' She continued to gaze into the dog's eyes. 'Could also be metaldehyde poisoning.'

I found a small degree of reassurance that Gemma was also somewhat perplexed as to the mystery toxin that had caused Bob's condition. I silently rattled through the list of toxic chemical compounds found in various known dog poisons: theobromine, chocolate; xylitol, chewing gum; warfarin, rodenticide; metaldehyde, slug pellets.

'At least if he *has* eaten a load of slug pellets, you'll know quickly,' Gemma continued. 'There'll be no mistaking it if his vomit comes out bright green or blue!'

Slug pellets, of course.

Ideally, we would induce vomiting with an injection. But making Bob vomit when he was already practically 'seizuring' was far too risky. Gastric lavage is the process of anaesthetising an animal in order to pass a tube down through the mouth, flush warm water into the stomach, then syphon it back out. The aim of this irrigation is to remove any potentially toxic ingesta before it has the chance to absorb further. It's only effective if the toxin was eaten within the past two hours. But as in Bob's case we had no idea *what* or indeed *when* the offending material was eaten, it was a balance between the risk of the procedure versus the benefit of removing further toxin.*

Using the line in his leg, I plunged the anaesthetic agent through the cannula and watched as Bob drifted into a calm and stationary restful sleep. His tremors ceased. He finally looked peaceful. Next, I passed an endotracheal tube down into his windpipe. Then we tilted the table so that his head was lower than his body, like a child about to launch head-first

---

* Nowadays there is conflicting evidence as to how useful the procedure of gastric lavage is if it isn't rapidly deployed after ingestion of an otherwise potent toxin, such as paracetamol in a cat. But still, if it is carried out carefully and with precaution, it's hopefully unlikely to worsen the situation and therefore is still considered a useful tool in the management of toxicity cases.

down a playground slide. I measured the distance from his mouth to his ribs and then passed the lubricated, soft rubber tip past his larynx, down the oesophagus and along the pre-measured length to his stomach. Warm water travelled up the tube from a bucket on the floor. Then the smell of his morning's partially digested breakfast filled the room as the watery, sludgey vomit trickled back down and out into a second bucket on the floor, like a sewage pipe draining the contents from the sleeping canine.

I repeatedly flushed clean water in, as the nurses gently palpated around his abdomen to help 'swill' the water around his stomach – like a washing machine on a gentle cycle – and then allowed it to trickle back into the waste bucket. Once the water that flowed from his stomach was as crystal clear as the water flowing in, I finished by administering a dose of activated charcoal. Knowing there was very little chance he would have the coordination to swallow for himself after recovering from the general anaesthetic, this was the best way to deposit the medicine directly into his stomach.

The jet-black charcoal paste slowly trickled down the stomach tube and coated his gastrointestinal tract, acting like a sponge and helping to mop up any of the remaining toxin that may still have been present in Bob's stomach. Then finally I folded the rubber tube to create a kink in the line and prevent any seepage of charcoal from the end that may otherwise risk causing an inhalation pneumonia, and with one swift action withdrew the tube from his mouth.

With the procedure finished I placed a glove onto my right hand and plunged it deep into the bucket of vomit. As I pulled a handful of gloopy, meaty brown debris, I looked to see if I could spot any of the offending turquoise green slug pellets. But there were none. Still we were none the wiser about what had caused his reaction.

As Bob slowly recovered from his anaesthetic and regained consciousness, his tremors gradually began to recur too. Of course, flushing his stomach may help, but that was never going to be the full cure. His blood screen results had all come back normal, but the question remained – what was wrong with him? And what should we do next?

As I stood waiting for Bob to continue his recovery, the receptionist hurriedly pushed through the prep room doors. 'James, Bob's owner is back in reception!' she said hurriedly. We all turned to look at her, listening closely over the beeping sound of the anaesthetic monitoring equipment. 'Her other dog is now starting to shake too. Can you come?'

The nursing team nodded their permission for me to leave Bob's side. I pulled the glove from my hand, threw it into the bucket and then followed her in a swift jog through to the reception area. Mrs Radford was standing in the middle of the room, wearing tracksuit bottoms and a comfortable hoody. I knew her well. She usually wore her hair in a straightened bob, with blonde streaks, blush lip gloss and hooped earrings. She always looked 'cool', for want of a better word. She favoured brightly coloured patterned dresses and paired them with comfortable trainers, usually with a sparkly silver Nike tick down the side. But not that day.

She was flushed, her eyes bloodshot red, tears streaming down her face, her hair greased back into a ponytail while her hands had imprinted a white powdery strike of flour across the front of her thighs thanks to a morning's attempt to bake a cake for her work colleagues. Her comfy morning of baking and self-care, a welcome break from her otherwise highly stressful job, had been suddenly interrupted by the mysterious onset of both her dogs developing a toxic reaction to an unknown substance.

'Oh my God, James . . .' she said hurriedly, through stifled tears, as I came through the doors. 'I think I've worked out what's happened!'

Her hands were shaking at almost the same rate and frequency as the little black scruffy dog encased in her arms. The dog was still conscious, but with a similar glazed look in her eyes and a continual shiver, with the occasional body-wide muscle spasm.

'I . . . I rushed out to the shop and . . . asked my h . . . husband to . . . to give the dogs their flea treatment,' she said as tears continued to well into her eyes. She carefully began to pass the second dog, Jill, over to me, then wiped her glistening tears from her red face with the palm of her right hand. 'B . . . but he just told me that h . . . he put it in their food instead of on their scruff.'

The words tripped out of her mouth as the guilt and realisation of what had happened washed over her. She pulled both her hands up to her head, pulled her fingers through her hair and looked at me with the panic of a mother in despair.

'Has he killed them?' she asked. 'Are they going to be OK?' she continued, in desperate need of reassurance. 'Oh my God, they'll be OK, won't they?'

Despite the written instructions on the packet, her husband had made the not entirely ridiculous presumption that the pipettes of liquid were designed to go on their food rather than their skin. He'd dosed each meal and then left for work. Thankfully, fate had pulled Mrs Radford home earlier than usual that day and she had found Bob shaking on the kitchen floor. I kept reassuring her that 'these things just happen'. But even as I uttered them, my words felt empty. There is little that can be said in these circumstances without sounding either horribly condescending or totally heartless. But accidents *do just* happen.

But what felt to Mrs Radford as a guilty confession, to me was the missing part of a clinical jigsaw puzzle. It was the clue I needed to begin tailoring our treatment for Bob and Jill. Now we finally knew what we were dealing with.

'Jill's so fussy with her food,' she said. 'So I'd be surprised if she's eaten that much. But Bob is a greedy little git. He'll often finish her food as well, if she leaves any, so I reckon he's probably had more.'

Only time would tell, but ingestion of ivermectin had a far more favourable outlook than slug pellet poisoning, which can rapidly prove fatal. I reassured her and she consented that we should do whatever was necessary to try to save them.

I took Jill through to the prep area and we treated her in a similar fashion: flushing her stomach under general anaesthetic, administering some charcoal and then supporting her – and Bob – with intravenous fluid therapy. Now with the knowledge of exactly what the toxin was, a separate drip line administered a lipid product – an infusion of white, liquid 'fat' – directly into the bloodstream to help absorb the toxin and allow the body to detoxify itself.

The two dogs lay side by side in adjoining kennels. Bags of saline and white lipid solution hung suspended from the drip stands on the outside of their kennels, with a transparent, soft, plastic line running underneath the metal grate door of each kennel and connected to the cannula port in each dog's leg. There was nothing more to do other than continually monitor their progress and regulate their temperature with cooling fans or warm heat pads if they dropped too low. Now we simply had to wait.

After a few hours of intensive nursing, Jill's tremors slowly dissipated and she began to regain consciousness. Bob took longer, having received a larger quantity of toxin after scoffing Jill's breakfast along with his own. But thankfully, with time, his tremors began to gradually ease as well. We kept the duo in the hospital overnight under the watchful gaze of the nursing team who stayed by their sides throughout. And then thankfully, the next day, both dogs made a full recovery and were able to be discharged to return home.

All this from a simple miscommunication between a husband and wife. In the end, no harm done, but in the heat of the moment, the guilt and shame across Mrs Radford's face were so vivid, I can still picture it now.

These kind of mishaps and encounters present themselves more frequently in a veterinary practice than you might think. Hindsight is a wonderful thing but looking after pets is an education in its own right – an education that builds with time. There is so much learning to be done. Sometimes that learning arrives through books or online, sometimes through your vets or vet nurses and sometimes from other pet owners passing on their knowledge. But sadly, sometimes learning comes the hard way – through the gaining of first-hand experience. With hindsight, of course, we would all change our actions, but sometimes all we can do is learn from our mistakes.

I'm not for one second suggesting we should be more flippant and not make every possible attempt to prevent an accident or illness from happening in the first place, but after fifteen years of myself having to counsel many pet owners through these very difficult and often tragic situations, I know only too well the pressure and judgement we all put on ourselves. And more often than not, that judgement comes mostly from within. As a fellow pet owner, I have made mistakes myself. And I have judged myself too. But our learning as pet parents never stops. This is a lesson I am all too familiar with.

CHAPTER 8

Oliver, Part II

I ran upstairs and scooped a fusty old gym T-shirt from the bedroom floor, then stepped both legs into my slouchy pair of tracksuit bottoms. I couldn't care less about my appearance. I just had to reach Oliver. I moved as fast as I physically could, my whole body trembling with adrenaline and fear. I grabbed the keys from the kitchen worktop and pushed both feet into a pair of trainers, then called for Mark to hurry and slammed the front door behind us. We both ran to the car.

As I clambered into the driver's side, I could see Mark's hands shaking as he sat braced in the passenger seat, his arms outstretched, both palms pressed flat against the dashboard. My mouth was dry. My heart was beating so hard and so fast I could feel it physically thumping from my chest to my throat. I turned the key and began to reverse the car from the driveway.

The words from the woman on the phone that Oliver was at least alive had offered some reassurance, but I knew if he was in shock, the adrenaline that pumped around his body could still have masked an underlying injury and everything could, at any point, take a turn for the worse. I felt the sudden awful realisation that there was a very high chance that in whatever state we might find him, Oliver may not survive.

Witnessing an animal in distress is always horrible. But for those working in the veterinary field, you somehow learn how to rationalise it. We spend every day reading our patients' behaviour, often in relation to pain. Our job is to respond, to counteract pain with the most appropriate level of pain relief, for example, and then set about fixing the underlying problem. We are equipped with the tools, the knowledge and the training to be able to help our animal patients. We can reduce their distress, take away their pain, or even end their suffering altogether. I believe there is something psychologically and perhaps subconsciously reassuring about knowing what to do and being able to help. We don't 'grow numb' but we learn to buffer our own emotional response to an animal in distress by coming up with a solution and utilising our skills to provide a physical response to help them.

My head and heart suddenly flooded with the worry that, while I had witnessed many animals presenting in various levels of trauma, Mark hadn't. He had recently returned from life in the French Alps running ski chalets and had never seen an animal covered with blood or crying in pain or at the end of life.

'There's a chance he might be in a really bad way when we get there,' I said quietly to him, as I hurled the car down the lane at breakneck speed. He nodded silently, his eyes wide and his gaze fixed on the road ahead. I also worried that I had no idea how I would respond. This was the first time in my years of being a vet that it had been my own pet who was suddenly in need of treatment. I hadn't a clue how I was going to react when I saw him. Would I be able to think rationally or would I fall to pieces?

It was only a few minutes past 6 a.m. and the sun was still rising. I could feel the adrenaline shooting around my blood-stream. I felt like I had injected a million shots of caffeine straight into my veins; my mind was racing, my heart was pounding, my hands were cold and I wanted to scream, cry and shout. But instead, I knew I just needed to drive. Stay focused. Find Oliver. And Jenson.

It was a dangerous road. The gently winding corners of the quiet country lane made it easy to pick up speed. A favourite course for the local bored teenagers in low cars with wide exhaust pipes and engines that sounded like a bunch of kids blowing raspberries against their own forearms. As a vet, it is fairly impossible to draw conclusions on the severity of trauma inflicted by a road traffic accident over the phone. Our response, as veterinary professionals, is to prioritise getting the pet to a vet practice as soon as possible. Until a patient has been fully assessed, it is very difficult to give a prognosis based on the 'first impressions' from an owner (unless, of course, it is the most catastrophic of cases).

We eventually reached the T-junction at the bottom of our lane. 'Left or right?' I asked, somewhat rhetorically as neither of us had a clue. Mark just looked at me in silence, his eyes filled with fear of what we might find.

'Try left,' he said intuitively. We took a chance. I turned the steering wheel and put my foot down. The gamble paid off. Moments later, I saw two cars pulled over with their hazard lights flashing. Instinct told me we had found them, but something deep inside me wished we could just keep going. Drive straight past. Suspend ourselves in time. That we wouldn't find Oliver because none of it was real. That he and Jenson would be jumping up at the kitchen door for their breakfast. That it had all just been a cruel hoax. A sick prank.

I edged the car closer and eventually pulled up to a halt. The clicking sound of the car's indicator counted as each agonising second ticked by, like a metronome keeping time on an orchestra about to crescendo. Then, between the two parked cars and nestled among the green and yellow dandelions of the roadside verge, I spotted a flash of Oliver's golden yellow coat. I killed the car's engine and we both hurried over.

A large grey 4x4 barricaded most of the verge. In front of the truck, a silver Ford Mondeo had also pulled over. There was a big dent over the front left wheel arch about the size, I'd hazard a guess, that a thirty-seven-kilogram Labrador could imprint. From between the two cars, the familiar female voice called out – it was the same neutral accent and warm-toned voice that had echoed around our bedroom walls only moments earlier. 'Over here!' she yelled, and raised her waving right arm up into the air. She wore a navy-blue polo-necked shirt with a white embroidered logo over the chest.

'Hi, I'm Georgie,' she called over from a crouched-down position in the grass verge and looked back over her shoulder at us. 'Are you the gents I spoke with?'

My head was muddled with shock and confusion. Georgie, though, remained calm, collected and in control. Reassuringly, she was everything I could *not* be at that time. 'Yes,' Mark replied. 'Thank you so much for calling us.'

We both clambered up the grass verge to where Georgie

143

was kneeling beside a big mound of golden fur. It was Oliver. 'Err, so, I think he's OK,' Georgie was quick to summarise. 'But I do think he's suffered a full radial fracture to his right forearm.' Reading the expression on both of our faces, she clarified her diagnosis with, 'It's OK, I'm a vet!' *Bloody hell, what are the chances?* I thought to myself. It was then that I noticed the logo on the side of the 4x4. Georgie was a farm animal vet. She had been driving past on her way home from an early dawn calving and pulled over to help.

Oliver's one chestnut-brown eye widened as his gaze met ours and his ears fell from a scared, tense triangular shape to a relaxed 'flop' that hung either side of his worried oval face. He lifted his head as he recognised our voices and pushed his nose forwards, as though trying to reach out and touch us. At the same time, his golden tail began to thud gently against the mound of grass in a slow, grateful, apologetic wag.

I knelt beside Georgie and smoothed both of his ears against his head. 'I'm so, so sorry.' I leant forwards and kissed the bridge of his nose. I looked up at Mark who had tears filling both his eyes. Both of us still searching our confused minds about how the two dogs had managed to escape in the first place and yet feeling the full weight of responsibility that we had completely failed not only Oliver, but Jenson too. Jenson. Where was Jenson?

With neither of us realising, a man had appeared next to Mark. He was dressed in a grey suit, had a white beard, grey metal oblong spectacle frames and a few strands of wispy white hair on the top of his balding head. And, as though in keeping with his monochrome style, his face and cheeks also looked white as a sheet. He was ashen, shaken, remorseful.

'It was me that hit him,' the man confessed. He spoke

quietly and still in a state of shock. 'The two of them, they just came running out from nowhere. I wasn't going fast but . . .' He stopped and stared at a patch on the road, his memory clearly playing over when and where the incident had played out.

'And I stopped to help,' he pointed to Oliver, 'but as I got out of the car the other one just ran off!' He spun on the spot, and looked around with both his arms raised to the side.

His tone was apologetic but with an undercurrent of frustration, perhaps even anger in his voice. He felt terrible that he had hit Oliver but clearly (and rightfully) he was more annoyed that they were on the loose, and out of control. He couldn't blame Oliver, but he did blame us. We had caused this, in his eyes. And he blamed us too for the fact he would have to live with the guilt of hitting a dog.

I wanted to question him. How fast he was driving? How could he not have seen such a huge yellow dog in the road? Was he on his phone? All the accusations came flooding to my mind – but instead, the guilt that Oliver was hurt took over. Deep down, I too blamed myself. 'I am just so, so sorry.' I turned to look at him. Mark echoed the apology.

The man was gentle, reserved; he looked like he'd never broken the speed limit in his life. We couldn't be angry. It was an accident. A series of unfortunate events that had led to the situation that we found ourselves in. Rather, we both began an uncontrollable torrent of apologies and 'thank yous' out of sheer gratitude to these two perfect strangers, eternally grateful that they had stopped and helped Oliver.

Having phoned the number she'd found on the silver tag that dangled from the one-eyed Labrador's collar, Georgie had used some towels and bandages from the calving kit in the boot of her truck to cover and shelter Oliver from the cool, wet dawn dew. Then placed a hefty dressing over the leg to help stabilise the fracture and comfort his pain. She offered to give me a hand to manoeuvre Oliver into the boot of my car.

We lifted him gently onto the makeshift stretcher of towels and moved him towards our car. In doing so he yelped out a high-pitched squeal. The gut-wrenching double 'halp' sound that dogs make when they feel in acute pain. And, with every yelp, it not only triggered within me a huge surge of guilt for the unimaginable pain that he was in. Guilt also that I had failed both dogs, that I hadn't protected them better and that I had massively let down Jenson's owner, Sarah.

We lowered his body into the boot of the car, swapped contact details and said our goodbyes. My intuition recognised that Oliver did at least seem critically stable. I kept everything crossed that we might escape this as nothing more than a fractured leg, but only time would tell. I needed to get him to the veterinary practice as soon as possible. But where was Jenson?

He couldn't be that far, Georgie had said. Yet we lived in rural Somerset – the main road was flanked by field after field after field. He could be anywhere. With Oliver safely cocooned in the boot of my car, we drove further along the road to see if we could spot any flashes of Jenson's dark brown and white markings in the sprawling green countryside around us.

My mind raced through every worst-case scenario imaginable.

We wound down the car windows and hollered Jenson's name. The roads were quiet and being out in the countryside,

I hoped our voices would travel far. Yet nothing. No sighting. No bark to be heard. No sign of Jenson anywhere. And worse, time was ticking. With Oliver in need of urgent medical attention, I knew that there was a limit to how long we could continue the search for Jenson. Worse still, I knew that Jenson was wearing a name tag similar to Oliver. What if someone else had already picked him up? What if they had already phoned Sarah? How would she feel finding out from a stranger that Jenson had gone missing? I knew what I had to do.

I listened to the ringtone, unsure of exactly what I should say, or how to explain the inexplicable. 'Hello, this is Sarah's phone. Please leave a message and I'll call you back.'

There was a long beep. Just long enough for me to make a split-second decision. Leave a message – how could I explain all this in a voicemail? Or hang up and risk someone else phoning her first. 'Oh, hi, Sarah,' I started. 'I'm really sorry to phone you on holiday, but ummm . . .' I paused, maybe a voicemail was not the right thing to do as I could hardly bring myself to say the words. 'Sadly we've had an accident this morning, and, errr, somehow Oliver and Jenson have managed to escape.'

I felt a sudden urge to hang up.

'Oliver's be-been hit by a car . . . erm . . .' – I swallowed hard, unsure of how to deliver the final cliffhanger detail – 'and, er, well, we haven't . . . we don't . . . we don't quite know where Jenson is . . . yet.'

The situation felt so much worse after saying it out loud.

'I just wanted to phone and give you the heads-up in case anyone dials your number from his tag. I'm so sorry. I'll keep you posted.'

I hung up. Probably the hardest phone call I have ever had to make in my entire life, and still to this day, I feel physically sick just recalling it.

With no sign of Jenson, we spun the car around and headed back towards the house. 'I'm going to have to get Oliver to work,' I said to Mark. 'Can you keep searching?'

Then, as we crawled along the main road, still calling Jenson's name out of the car windows, a lady appeared at the bottom of her driveway. A huge mansion house, with large wooden gates, only a hundred yards from where Oliver's accident had happened. She wore a pale blue and baby pink striped rugby shirt and a pair of dark navy cotton trousers. A huge nest of blonde hair wobbled on the top of her head as she waved ferociously at us. 'HERE! OVER HERE!' she shouted over to us.

We pulled into the layby that led to her driveway and we both jumped out of the car. 'Have you lost a dog?' she shouted over to us as we hurried along the gravelled layby to reach her.

Running towards her in an unkempt, exhausted, budget version of the slow-motion *Baywatch* run, puffing and panting with each shuffle and stride, I shouted, 'Oh my God, is he dead?' All tremendously dramatic.

'Oh, for goodness' sake, no! He's right as rain. I found him playing with my two in the orchard!' She spoke in a hurried, upper England kind of way. 'He's a nice lad. Will you breed? Is he a stud? I noticed he's still got his tackle.'

'Oh my God, thank you!'

I flung both my arms around her neck as though I had just been rescued from a desert island. 'Thank you, thank you.' I hugged and hugged her.

'Oh, not to worry!' she replied, giving me three firm pats on my back, as if to say, 'Please let go of me.'

Mark explained the situation, that we had Oliver in the car with a broken leg.

'Oh, bloody hell!' the woman replied. 'You must go. Go now. Keep that lead.' She pointed to the slip lead around Jenson's neck. 'I've got hundreds. Good luck!' She waved her hand again in the air and walked back up her driveway.

'I'll walk him home,' Mark said, 'just phone me later.' He reached into the car and stroked Oliver on the head and told him he loved him.

With Jenson safely on his way back home with Mark, I heard Oliver whimper as he tried to find a comfortable position for his broken leg. I climbed back into the driver's seat and restarted the engine. My mind refocused on Oliver, and I realised there was no time to waste. I had to get him to the practice. Only then could I work out what had happened. And more importantly, what I needed to do to make it all better.

CHAPTER 9

Lenny

Julian, the head vet from a nearby zoo, had arrived to deliver a presentation to all the large animal farm and equine vets. He assembled the projector and angled it towards the wall of the staffroom, adjusted the aperture size and then cranked the dial so the title slide came into focus. His presentation was on elephant reproduction.

It began with a grainy black and white diagram of an elephant's reproductive tract. The next slide depicted the changing shape of a developing elephant foetus at various gestational stages over a twenty-two-month period (the length of time it takes to grow from an elephant embryo to a fully fledged calf). And finally, Julian explained the range of specific signs the keepers were looking for: increased activity, increased urination or defecation, mammary development and the production of milk, and the beating of the elephant's vulva with her tail, all tell-tale early signs that the first stage of labour had begun and that at some point in the next several days a baby elephant was soon on its way.

He loaded some video footage that had been captured on the zoo's CCTV of an elephant birth in the early stages of labour from three years previously. After a minute or two of rocking forwards and backwards, the mother elephant then crouched slightly, shifted her weight from side to side on her back feet, then flicked her tail. Suddenly, like a river bursting through a dam, several bucket loads of amniotic fluid came gushing from her back end. Through the cascading waterfall of clear, blood-tinged liquid, an infant elephant came tumbling along, expelled within seconds, and deposited onto a straw bed below. The zookeepers then pulled the newborn elephant to one side, covered it with towels and rubbed vigorously. Through their coordinated effort they revived and welcomed the newborn to the outside world. Next a stethoscope was placed against the chest wall, swabs were taken from her mouth, her eyes checked with an ophthalmoscope and then eventually the neonate was presented back to her mother for continued care.

Standing with an M&S sandwich in one hand, in front of a room of twenty or so gawping farm and equine vets (myself included), the zoo vet hit fast-forward on the remote control. He swallowed hard on his mistimed bite of sandwich. 'So, that would be the perfect birth in our eyes,' he said, holding up the sandwich to the screen.

The timer in the bottom right corner of the screen zoomed rapidly through approximately seventy minutes or so, and then he hit play again. The newborn elephant was by then standing and already searching with her trunk for her mother's teat. The room was electric. Everyone started commenting to each other: 'Woah, that's amazing!' 'No way!' 'That's so cool!'

The zoo vet took a moment. He soaked up the enthusiasm in the room and the collective smiles on everyone's faces. The room hushed, and he continued: 'OK, so if that video showed the perfect birth, the question is, what if something goes wrong? And that is where you guys come in.' He flashed a glance across to the four partners of the practice grinning like schoolkids.

'In the coming weeks we are expecting another elephant birth,' Julian continued, 'and we're asking for you to be on standby, in case we need a helping hand.' The look on the partners' faces suggested this was a done deal.

The mood shifted slightly. Some colleagues clearly relished the challenge of being pushed beyond their boundaries, to dip their toe in the world of zoological veterinary practice. Others immediately recognised how preposterous this seemed – an elephant under the responsibility of a horse vet posed a significant chance that things could go completely tits up, resulting in the inevitable witch hunt to find *someone* to blame (probably the equine vet, with no qualifications whatsoever to be treating an elephant in the first place).

'Don't worry, we get that this may sound like a strange request. But in zoo practice, the reality is, we just don't see that many births – whereas you guys, in domestic and farm practice, have far more experience. So really we see it as a kind of joining of forces.'

He sounded convincing. He continued to explain that the reproductive tract of the elephant is very similar to that of the horse, so it had been agreed that the equine vets (including myself) would be first on call. But the farm vets had more experience in reproductive medicine, so we should all be briefed as any one of us may be called upon to help.

'Now, before you ask, no, we do not expect you to perform a caesarean section on an elephant!' Julian explained. A few chuckles erupted around the room. 'Of the very few attempted elephant caesareans, they have all invariably proved fatal for both the mother elephant and her calf, so generally speaking, we don't really consider that an option.'

That put to bed the vision in my head of performing surgery with a bread knife and a forklift truck. Furthermore, he had explained, oxytocin must be used with extreme caution as the elephant womb could rupture if the cervix hasn't fully dilated.

'The reason we need you on backup is that I'm going away for three weeks on annual leave at the end of the month and so I won't be around. We're hoping, if all goes to plan, she'll give birth within the next fortnight, but it would be great to know we have some extra support should we need it in an emergency,' he concluded.

As Julian finished his sarnie, there was some nervous applause from his newly recruited (if reluctant) elephant army and then he left. No one really knew what exactly it was we had just signed up for, but the partners of the practice offered at least some reassurance that this would be a team effort. And so began the weeks of nervous waiting. It may sound enticing, challenging, a rare opportunity to work with elephants. And of course, it would have been. But with none of us having any elephant experience under our collective veterinary belts, with every day that ticked by, we all felt a shared sense of mild dread that we may be 'the one' to get called at 2 a.m. to aid an elephant with birthing difficulties.

There is an undercurrent of fear I've noticed among a lot of vets, especially younger or more recently qualified vets, that any mistake – no matter how small, whether defensible or not – will result in them being immediately struck off and given the boot without fair trial. This fear is particularly heightened when faced with new challenges or pushed outside of one's own 'clinical comfort zone'. And I can remember at that point in my career, I certainly felt that fear.

Of course, it's exactly right prevent reckless or dangerous practice and to hold the profession to account. But it can sometimes feel as though veterinary medicine has changed so much from the days of 'have a go and do your best' to 'on your head be it'. So even though the idea of treating a baby elephant sounds incredibly exciting, when faced with the reality, 'the fear' meant the team weren't exactly forthcoming in their enthusiasm.

We all left the meeting with mixed feelings, and reluctantly resumed our afternoon call-outs. Nothing else particularly spectacular happened that Friday. I worked through the vaccination appointments, I picked up a couple of extra calls in the afternoon, I stopped mid-afternoon and opened the boot of my car to let Oliver have a good stretch across some farmers' fields (he travelled around with me in the day) and I even managed to grab an afternoon coffee on the drive, a much-needed caffeine hit to help me power through the remaining afternoon.

A week or so after Julian's presentation, an internal email pinged up on my computer:

Polite reminder: this weekend all farm and equine partners will be at Julie's wedding in Amsterdam, with the exception of Megan who is on call for farm, and James for equine. Under these exceptional circumstances with all staff and partners away at

*once, Mike from the small animal hospital will be
contactable in case of emergency. And finally, we all
wish Julie our congratulations on her wedding day.*

I picked up the on-call pager from the desk and listened to
each of my colleagues as they delivered their half-hearted
apologies that I couldn't join them on their trip to Amsterdam.
With that, my weekend on call began. It was a surprisingly
quiet Saturday morning. 'Quiet' is a banned word in most
veterinary practices, the superstition being that the moment
someone utters the 'Q' word, the phone will start ringing. But
not that day. I even managed to go out for dinner that evening
with Mark, who by then had grown increasingly tired of trying
to book anything around the many nights or weekends I was
on call. Another dinner alone in a pub or restaurant could be
the final straw. So, generally speaking, and for the sake of our
relationship, we had stopped tempting fate.

At 8.30 a.m. on the Sunday morning I went to check on
the inpatients. The equine hospital was located at the rear of
the farm animal practice. An impressive set-up boasting ten
stable blocks, a large sand-floored manège (training area),
stalls to perform endoscopies, a weigh bridge to accurately
determine the weight of a horse in kilograms, an operating
theatre and a padded 'knock-down box' to safely anaesthe-
tise the equine patients. Unusually, I had only two inpatients
that weekend. Normally the stables would be at capacity at
the weekends, and it could easily take a whole morning just
to get through all the check-ups, working out and drawing up
of medications, bandage changes, cannula placements and
repeat clinical re-examinations.

But this particular weekend there were just two. The first

was a stunning grey mare that had been hospitalised after sinus surgery to relieve an infection that had brewed in the large, cavernous air-filled sinus spaces in her head. Each space that should be occupied by air had instead filled with thick, yellow, custard pus. A trephined hole had been created through her forehead, into which some tubing had been fed and the contents of a bucket of warmed saline solution could be flushed to irrigate the infected cavity. I pumped the grey handle of the gardener's spray gun, the type that more usually would be used to spray roses or feed the tomatoes in a greenhouse, but also created the perfect pressure to syphon saline solution into a horse's head, against gravity, to flush a snotty sinus. The saline filled the cavity and successfully out-competed the pus for space. A deluge of thick, yellow pus came pouring out of the horse's nostrils before glooping into a diluted mess on the floor, like toothpaste in the sink after being mixed with saliva and water. Surprisingly, horses often tend to tolerate this procedure pretty well.

For this mare, though, it was the trickling sensation down her face she enjoyed the least, throwing her head up and down without warning, as she flicked the saline-diluted pus into the air, showering both myself and the equine nurse on call with me. Midway through the final pump, I heard the pager vibrate on the table next to us. 'Aaaaagh,' I grumbled, 'I'd better get that, sorry.' I disconnected my gardener's pump and pulled the soft rubber tubing from the hole in the mare's head. I turned to retrieve the pager but, as I looked up, I noticed several flecks of yellow, cottage cheese pus had splattered through the nurse's otherwise deep chestnut-brown locks of hair.

'You've just got a little . . .' I smirked, and wiggled my

finger to the small section of fringe she had pulled across her forehead.

'Oh, shut up!' she replied, smiling. 'You don't look much better yerself!' she fought back, then laughed in a way that asked, 'Why *did* we chose this career?' A fair enough question to ask as the two of us were covered with horse snot on a Sunday morning.

I pulled the pager from its case and checked the screen. I read the words. And then read the words again. And then my heart sank.

'You've got to be ffffffff-lipping kidding me,' I said out loud as I read the message.

'What is it?' the nurse called over, teasing the clumps of cottage cheese pus from the strands of her fringe.

'Two-day-old elephant. Neurological problems. Please call zoo immediately,' I read aloud.

Before the whole veterinary team had left for Amsterdam, a second internal email had popped up on the Friday afternoon, addressed to all equine and farm vets in the practice:

GOOD NEWS – we have just heard from the zoo, elephant born safely last night! All went well. Can all stand down and breathe a sigh of relief!

But now I had this new message on my pager.

'Oh God!' the nurse replied, and looked at me with a genuinely concerned look of sympathy written all over her face.

We had been primed to help with the elephant birth, but I hadn't quite envisaged that might extend into the care of the neonate. Understanding the elephant birthing process sounded complicated enough. How to even begin navigating the topic of elephant neonatal neurology was completely mind-boggling.

'I'll have to go.' I wiped down my hands and arms in the clean bucket of diluted iodine.

'You might wanna check in the mirror before you set off!' the nurse replied, this time with a seriousness and cautious empathy that my veterinary skills were about to be fully tested to their very limit.

I smiled in an attempt to suppress the nervous volcano of worry that had filled the pit of my stomach. Then I knelt by a bucket and plunged my cupped hands deep into some diluted iodine solution, threw the medicinal diluent all over my face, spitting through my wet lips as I refilled my hands and repeated the face wash.

'I've got no idea what this is going to be or how long it'll take. Are you OK to finish up with the inpatients? Just call me if you have any worries,' I said to the nurse, aware that time was against me.

'Yeah, of course,' she replied.

I grabbed my keys, wiped down my hands, arms (and face) and jumped in the car.

As I reached the zoo, a queue of Sunday tourists had already started to snake their way around the car park. It was the middle of August, the school summer holidays, and an acne-fied teenager in the ticket booth waved me through. I drove my car slowly past the raised red and white barrier and followed in the trail of the zoo's logo – emblazoned on the side of a green quad bike.

The parents with young children slowly moved to the side as we crept through the crowds, working our way along the gently meandering path that led us towards the elephant enclosure. Eventually, we pulled up to a layby outside some brown wooden buildings with the words 'Laboratory' and 'Staff only' on each door. I collected together a handful of veterinary equipment from the back seat of my car – some gloves, a stethoscope, a thermometer – and threw them in my examination box and we continued the remainder of our trail on foot.

As we walked, parents knelt beside their children and pointed at us, smiling as we made our way through the final pedestrianised zones. 'Oooh, Look! It's the vet,' I heard one parent explain. 'He's come to make the poorly animals better.' I smiled. The young mother smiled back while the toddler stared at us in bewilderment. Being personally escorted through the public spaces all felt very 'important' but also served as a reminder of the enormous pressure I was under. And while I had dedicated plenty of headspace to how the hell I was going to treat a baby elephant, I had totally overlooked the fact that there would be an audience of tourists around. Hundreds of paying customers, poised, eager to catch a rare glimpse of some live veterinary drama. I could feel their eyes watch my every move – ready to judge, photograph and, even worse, *video record* my unrehearsed, impromptu and very much off-the-cuff performance of *How to Bluff Your Way Through Being an Elephant Vet*.

Thankfully, the path eventually quietened. Traffic cones were placed strategically across the width of the path, joined together with red and white plastic tape that had been looped around the tip of each cone. A laminated sign dangled from the plastic tape: 'NEW ARRIVAL!! To keep stress to a minimum, we have temporarily closed the elephant enclosure, but please keep an eye on our Facebook page for daily updates. Thank you.'

We both stepped over the tape and the crowds melted away behind us. But as we neared the main viewing platform, my guide suddenly deviated off the tourist path and led me towards a door with a sign that read 'PRIVATE – NO ENTRY'.

He punched in a code to the metal keypad on the heavy, forest-green door, twisted the latch sharply to the right, then heaved it open. 'Come in, through here.'

I felt hugely privileged. If I could tell my thirteen-year-old self that one day I would be behind the scenes in one of the UK's leading zoos about to come face to face with a forty-eight-hour-old elephant calf, I would never have believed it. Yet here I was. However, rather than dwell on childhood dreams, I had a job to do. And that brief feeling of privilege quickly changed to an overwhelming sense of responsibility.

'Just, like, stay here,' the young lad awkwardly insisted. 'Martha won't be long.' He then exited through the same door.

Martha was the head zookeeper. She must have left instructions to deposit me in that precise location, as the lad seemed both terrified of her and adamant that I must not move. The room was small, with a chest freezer at one end and a poster with antibiotic drug doses pinned on the wall above. There was a small desk with a number of books and boxes stacked beneath it and another door at the end of this corridor office with a glass window at head height. I guessed I was standing in Julian's office.

I reverted to feeling like a student on work experience. Standing, waiting for someone more important than myself to arrive and tell me what to do, where to stand and when to speak. Except this time, I would need to do more than just observe.

All of a sudden, a mop of curly, wiry, jet-black hair appeared at the window. The door latch turned, and the door opened just a few inches.

'NOT THERE!' her voice boomed. I jumped. Me? Was she referring to me? She opened the door further. She was talking over her shoulder, shouting towards someone a lot further away.

She spun her head round and stepped fully through the door, allowing it to slowly shut behind her. Her face was weathered, her pale complexion made all the more translucent against the bottle-dyed black perm. Her eyes looked as though she hadn't slept in days – which, I guessed, she probably hadn't. A short-sleeved, buttoned-up khaki shirt encased her bosom, the zoo's logo on her right and the name 'MARTHA VAN HEERDEN' embroidered underneath. Her shirt was tucked neatly into a pair of muddy green cargo shorts, and her thighs narrowed to a pair of dark brown laced-up leather boots. A thick leather belt wrapped around her waist helped to delineate where the shirt stopped and the shorts started and a black walkie-talkie hung on her right hip, clipped to the belt.

'Are you the vet they've sent?' she asked. A thick South African accent added to her already stern, intimidating presence.

'I am. Hi, I'm James,' I replied.

She looked me up and down. The last vague remnants of horse pus in my spiked fringe probably didn't cast a brilliant first impression. Nor the glistening snail trail of dried snot across the right shoulder of my navy-blue polo shirt where

the mare had managed to wipe her nose on me, just before
I'd left.

'Right,' she said. 'How long have you been qualified?'

'Err, it'll be three and a half years now,' I replied with de-
fiance, to make it sound like the number had no significance
on my overall capability to handle whatever she was hiding
behind that door. Of course, though, I immediately clocked
the disappointment in her eyes.

'OK, well, you'd better come through here.'

She reopened the door and we both stepped into the next
room. Immediately, the punchy smell of elephant dung filled
the air. Not quite as sweet as the smell of horse manure, but
far more intense.

We walked along a short corridor. After a few paces, the
wall to my left suddenly ended. The solid concrete passage-
way disappeared and was replaced instead with thick metal
bars that ran from floor to ceiling, spaced roughly about a
foot apart from each other. The walkie-talkie on Martha's hip
started spluttering. The scratchy, muffled voice spoke far too
quickly; neither of us could hear or decipher any meaningful
sentence. Martha stopped abruptly. She huffed, unclipped
the walkie-talkie, excused herself and took a few paces away
from me to explain – once again – that someone had to talk
'much ... *slower* ... please' through the radio.

With Martha preoccupied, I stood and faced the enclosure.
I placed both hands on two of the bars and leant my head
slightly forwards. Between the metal poles, in the distance
and slightly tucked around the corner I saw the adult Asian
elephant, the closest I had ever been to such a huge, magnificent animal. I watched as she lifted her trunk in response
to a cue from her designated handler, who I presumed was

162

the person Martha had shouted at. With each lift of her trunk, the handler placed an apple into the elephant's open mouth. Then, with Mum preoccupied, from underneath her emerged a perfectly formed baby elephant, an exact miniature replica of her adult self, trotting around in between his mother's legs.

No more than three or four feet tall, his grey wrinkly skin mottled with tiny salmon pink blotches made him desperately cute and surprisingly hairy! The baby elephant wandered, one foot in front of the other, away from his mother, and in my direction. I observed his movements. He seemed quite co-ordinated initially, then suddenly his front right foot caught short and he stumbled forwards. His left foot reacted quickly enough to prevent him tumbling completely, but as soon as his stride recovered, he was aimlessly wandering once more. He walked slowly, more of a plod, dragging his feet in no particular direction. For want of a better word, he looked sozzled! As though he'd sunk ten pints down the local boozer and been told to walk home. Even with my limited experience of elephants specifically, it was abnormal to witness a young mammal wander so far from its mother, without purpose, without fear, and for no reason. As her offspring aimlessly walked further away, the mother elephant turned to watch, but with two of her legs tethered, connected by metal chains to large hoops cemented into the floor, all she could do was let out the most almighty high-pitched blast, like a foghorn sounding through a thousand megaphones. The sound shuddered around the huge indoor enclosure.

'WHAT THE HELL ARE YOU DOING?' Martha's voice boomed from behind as she raced forwards and smacked her walkie-talkie against the galvanised metal bar. The loud 'clang' reverberated the full length of the metal pole from floor to ceiling and back again. I stepped back and stared at her, unsure of quite what I had done so wrong. 'Do not ever put your head, or your arm, or your hand, or anything through these bars ever again or you are out of here!' She tapped her walkie-talkie repeatedly against the bar as she listed off each body part.

'OK . . . OK . . . I'm . . . I'm sorry.' I quickly moved away from the bars, a little baffled.

She pointed her arm out to the adult elephant in the distance, careful to keep her arm *on our side* of the bars. 'One swing of that trunk at full speed and you will be decapitated!'

My eyes widened. 'My God,' I replied.

'Yah. No joke. And I'm not exaggerating.' She pointed her walkie-talkie at me, as though she was telling off a child.

I felt the seriousness in her voice.

'These are not pets, they are not domesticated animals, this is not a farm and you are not at the circus,' she said over her shoulder towards me as she simultaneously buckled the walkie-talkie back onto her belt. 'This is a conservation zoo.' We set off again and continued our walk along the corridor. I followed Martha as she picked up pace.

'These animals play a vital contribution to the endangered species zoo breeding programme. The way we manage them means they still possess the natural instincts and behaviours you may encounter in the wild – so from now, you follow my every direction extremely closely.'

I nodded.

'This way.' She directed me with her arm round a sharp corner.

We followed the metal bars into a second tunnel of solid

concrete walls that opened up once more into a much larger space. The same metal bars separated this room from the main elephant enclosure. It all felt quite penal, as though the natural physical strength of the elephant was also somehow her crime, with her feet being tethered and her life behind bars. I admired the conservation aspect but did question in my mind how closely the life of these animals could be compared to their wild counterparts. The room was equipped with tables, buckets of chopped vegetables, a huge hosepipe, multiple yard brooms and a gate through the metal bars to allow a human to enter or exit the enclosure.

'OK, here he is.' She spoke quietly, and pointed over to the wandering elephant calf.

He was circling, slowly shuffling round and round without any purpose or clarity, like a lost driver on a roundabout unsure of which direction to take. *Where do I even start?* I thought to myself. Neurology is a hugely complex area of veterinary medicine and often relies on advanced imaging such as an MRI or CT scan to fully diagnose the underlying concern. But there was only me, and my stethoscope, and a team of hopeful zoo workers all staring at my blank face.

'Right,' I said, 'can I take a closer look?' I picked up the examination case and looked to Martha for permission.

'What do you want to look at?' Martha replied, keeping a fixed stare on the baby elephant and avoiding my eyeline completely.

'Well, I'll need to perform a clinical exam!' I replied, somewhat bemused.

'What, though? What is it you need to examine? Talk me through *exactly* what you're planning to do.'

'Well, as much as feasibly possible: heart rate, temperature, cranial nerves, reflexes . . .'

Martha remained silent. I sensed her distrust in me.

'I will need to examine him,' I said quietly, 'if I'm going to have any chance of working out what's going on!'

Her silence continued. 'I do not want to cause any undue stress to these animals,' she said eventually. 'Those chains around her feet are a last resort. I do not tether the animals under my care unless we are in exceptional circumstances.' She looked at me. 'And these are exceptional circumstances.' She held her stare to ensure I had recognised the seriousness of the situation.

'I cannot tell you how she'll react, but I can tell you she will find us approaching her calf extremely stressful. Jack and Sal, you go with James, please. EVERYONE, please remain alert, and NOBODY is to approach the mother.'

The team nodded.

'OK, let him in.'

I stepped through the gate into the enclosure. The enormity of the situation hit. To be in the same space as one of the world's most gigantic, powerful and beautifully intelligent animals, with no physical boundary between us, felt both intimidating and thrilling in equal measure. Jack and Sal were two of the keepers. They had both been working around the clock from the days that led up to the birth and ever since. They led me quietly over to the youngster, who was still stuck on his merry-go-round, walking in circles.

The two of them stepped close and with joint arms managed to slow his walking to a stop. However, despite the neurological challenges, he was sufficiently conscious to understand that we had approached, and he began to panic. He pushed forwards, like the prop in a rugby scrum, to escape the joint clutches of the two keepers, but this wasn't their first meeting. The keepers were skilled. In a coordinated, collective effort, they kept their locked arms together and followed the young elephant, allowing him to reach a corner of the enclosure where he eventually came to a standstill and surrendered.

They stood with a wide-legged stance, knees slightly bent and their torsos pressed into the infant elephant's shoulder. Sal looked over at me. 'OK, you can come and look at him now!' she called.

I walked slowly over to his left side. I placed my veterinary examination box on the ground and unclipped the two metal latches, then lifted the lid to reveal a variety of diagnostic instruments. 'All right,' I said, 'let's start with his heart rate.'

I placed the soft rubber buds into my ear canals. The outside world was temporarily silenced. I tapped the drum of the stethoscope and felt the two pings travel up to my ears. I placed my right hand onto the withers of the elephant, and holding the drum of the stethoscope in my left, I lowered it to his chest. A deep thudding sound penetrated through the chest wall and along the rubber tube of my stethoscope. I counted the beats. I felt my hand on the elephant's shoulder, the firm bristles and his rough, creviced skin. I moved the stethoscope over his chest and listened to both his heart and lung sounds. Then further back again, to listen over his abdomen.

I shone the bright light of an ophthalmoscope into each of the eyes, and the periocular wrinkled skin contracted as he tried to close his eyelids. I prised them open gently with my thumb and forefinger and watched as the piercing pupil constricted, as expected, in response to the bright light. I lifted his tail and took a temperature reading. I checked the tip of his trunk for any discharge. I felt along the curvature of his spine and lifted each foot in turn to ensure there was no restriction to the joint movement, or the crunching sensation of bone fracture. Nothing. Everything appeared normal. Except for his general state of mental dullness and incoordination.

Sweat began to collect on my brow and upper lip. Five minutes of clinical examination with nothing to report other than the obvious neurological signs. How could I go back to Martha with no diagnosis? 'OK, thanks. I think we can probably let him relax for a while again,' I said to the keepers, whose backs were just about to collapse under the strain of maintaining a flexed restraint against 100 kg of solid muscle.

We walked back through the gate and Martha looked at me. 'Well?'

'All his vital parameters seem pretty normal – so this *is* most likely to be neurological.'

'And what does that mean?' She looked at me expectantly.

'Well, it means I can't tell you *exactly* what this is on exam alone,' I said, disappointingly.

She turned her head away. I placed the toolkit down on the table and scrambled through my thoughts. I knew I could do better. Then, a flash of inspiration. I turned to Martha. 'How did the actual birth itself go?' I asked. 'Do you have any CCTV footage I could take a look at?'

Martha led me back to the original office. She pulled back the chair from under the desk and retrieved a laptop from the top drawer of a filing cabinet. After a few minutes, she clicked onto a file that had the date from two days previously.

A grainy video loaded, and Martha moved the cursor so the image filled the screen. 'OK, here you go.' She leant back in the chair. 'There's nothing much to see.'

The video played out. True to Martha's word, there was nothing particularly abnormal. It followed pretty much the exact same sequence of events that we had witnessed in Julian's presentation. The young elephant came shooting out in a torrent of fluid, in similar fashion to the one we saw in the meeting – he tumbled to the ground, the team resuscitated him, then he stood and after half an hour or so he started to search for his mother's teat.

'And how long did that take?' I asked Martha. 'The actual birth? All the way from first stage to delivery?'

'Hmmm.' Martha leant forwards and used the cursor to scroll rapidly through the video's timeline, moving forwards and back, searching for the key events and noting down the timings. 'I'm going to say maybe twelve hours, max?' she concluded. 'To be honest, we normally expect the first stage of labour to last at least a few days or so, but as soon as she'd started, it was all over.'

'So, you'd say, in your experience, it was a pretty quick process?' I asked.

'Yah, she just pushed him straight out!'

Bingo. 'I wonder if that might have something to do with it,' I replied.

Martha listened silently. I pointed at the laptop screen. 'That seemed like a much speedier birthing process than the one Julian described. Whether or not it is even a recognised condition in elephants, I've no idea, but his symptoms follow pretty much the *exact* same pattern as a foal with neonatal maladjustment syndrome* – the "dummy foals", as they're known, start off normal, but progress to develop neurological issues after only a few hours or days.'

She nodded and looked at the computer screen.

'Is it possible to take a blood sample?' I asked.

She took some convincing, but with Martha reluctantly on board, I stepped back into the enclosure with the two keepers. The baby elephant's floppy earlobe, the size of a dinner plate, wafted like a huge leaf of an exotic tree. He flapped the ear out of my hand a number of times, with an incredible strength. Eventually, though, Sal managed to hold the ear still. She restrained his body with her knee as I swabbed the skin with surgical spirit. A huge vein ran along the peripheral margin of the ear. Martha's last piece of advice: 'The vein will look huge through the skin, but the actual vessel is only about the size of a strand of spaghetti. It is VERY difficult to get a sample. Please, only one attempt but no more or you will cause too much trauma.'

---

* Nobody really knows the exact cause of neonatal maladjustment syndrome. It affects roughly 1–2 per cent of newborn foals and is linked to early placental separation, reduced oxygenation and rapid birth deliveries. It is believed there is a failure to 'switch off' the neurosteroids that keep a foal relatively still in the womb. These neurosteroids prevent the foal from moving around too much, which could otherwise damage the uterus. However, as the neurosteroids remain, the foal never really fully reaches wakefulness. They are disorientated and confused – a so-called 'dummy' foal. The treatment in foals is largely supportive. The 'foal squeeze' is also sometimes applied – whereby a set of ropes is applied around the foal's chest to 'swaddle' them for twenty minutes, to replicate the passage through the birth canal, and this is now recognised as a valuable step in treating these foals. However, this technique had not been discovered at the time.

She was not wrong. I lined up the needle and inserted it directly into the centre of the hosepipe-sized vein, but no blood. I could feel and see the vein beautifully clearly, but even after I gently redirected the needle tip, still nothing. Knowing this was my only attempt, I forced the needle with a rapid 'stab' in case the vein was evading puncture and then I saw it – a small amount of blood flashed into the needle hub. I withdrew the plunger and thick, maroon-red liquid filled the first centimetre of the syringe. It wasn't much, but it was enough.

'Great! Thank you,' I said, signalling to Sal to keep some light pressure on the site for a minute or so.

I walked back to the gate and as I did so, the infant released a small blow through his trumpet. It was quiet, but even to the human ear it sounded like a distress call. The mother turned, her feet rattling the chains, and released a sound that made every surface in the enclosure vibrate.

Martha shouted through the bars, 'RELEASE HIM!'

The infant elephant immediately escaped the embrace of the two keepers and managed to coordinate enough strides to reunite himself with his mother.

We all stepped through the gate and closed the bars behind us. Back in the safety of the keepers' area Martha explained to her team that no one was to re-enter the enclosure for at least an hour. She turned to look at me, tilted her head forwards and looked over the bridge of her nose: 'That's it. No more.'

I placed a few drops of blood onto the handheld glucometer and allowed the rest to fill two capillary tubes to take a PCV reading. 'He's becoming dehydrated,' I said, 'and his sugar levels are dropping.

'Can we phone Julian?' I asked, hoping to run my findings past him and see if he had any preference on how we should proceed.

Martha turned and glared at me. 'Absolutely not,' she replied.

Her tone suggested that this was not even up for debate. Apparently, Julian had made it crystal clear that *no one* was to contact him while he was on annual leave, even in an emergency.

I was starting to feel quite frustrated. How and why was I alone in this situation? In my mind, this elephant was surely a vitally important member of the zoo's inhabitants? Their history? Their success? There had to be someone else they could call upon, a vet from another zoo? Or someone with elephant experience perhaps? Someone who could advise properly on what to do next. I could not carry the weight of this elephant on my own shoulders, surely?

It was time to put the cards on the table. 'OK, well, all I can say is this: if he was a foal, I would now suggest he be hospitalised for intensive care treatment. We'd be doing regular blood analysis, he would be on supplementary intravenous support, possibly require a plasma transfusion. He'd need around-the-clock feeds and constant monitoring for at least seven, maybe up to ten days.'

Martha listened as I delivered my verdict.

'It is a complicated diagnosis, but with correct treatment, in a foal the prognosis would be pretty good.'

I tried to sound professional but inwardly I felt as though I was on trial. I could only extrapolate from my equine knowledge, but I was fully aware it could be completely different when applied to elephant medicine. I was partly talking science and partly guessing. 'The treatment is large-ly supportive and that's even *if* we've reached the correct diagnosis,' I said with hesitation and growing concern. 'But I really just don't know what more to say or do from here.'

She looked at me quizzically.

'His life will be hanging on a knife edge if we don't support him through the next few days,' I said to Martha.

The pressure and enormity of the situation seemed to finally sink into her face. Perhaps she hadn't quite expected me to wave my white flag and ask for help, but I had noth-ing left to offer. Yet still, she remained silent. Clearly, being fobbed off with a junior horse vet had been nothing short of an insult to her elephant breeding programme in their time of need. Perhaps Julian had overpromised to his zoological coworkers and colleagues about the veterinary support he had arranged in his absence. Perhaps our practice partners had underdelivered on their promise. I'd never know. But with Julian in the Maldives and my colleagues all in Amster-dam, I was all there was available. Despite the humiliation in that moment, I knew there was a finite amount of time the elephant had left alive unless *someone* intervened on a pretty mammoth scale.

'I have already made contact with another zoo vet,' Martha confessed coldly, but with a tone that suggested she recognised I was slowly sinking.

'GOOD!' I replied. The relief. Humiliation aside, I just wanted someone, *anyone*, to help me or tell me what to do.

Shortly after, a phone call came through. The elephant vet spoke with fluent accuracy, an American slant to her international accent as we conversed on speaker phone in the elephant enclosure. I explained the symptoms. She suggested that, as with any neonate, nutrition and supportive measures would be the key to survival in the short term. She talked me through how to administer some emergency fluid therapy and advised we started him on oral antibiotics that I luckily had in the car and could leave with Martha. The vet had already booked her flight and would arrive in the UK from Europe in around fourteen hours' time.

Fourteen hours, I thought to myself. Just fourteen more hours that I needed to keep the elephant alive for and then I could hand the reins over to the international elephant expert who was flying in to save the day. Fourteen out of only eighteen hours left of being on call – just one more night to get through, to hope that no more emergency calls would land, and to hopefully get some rest before 9 a.m. on Monday morning, when another full working week would begin.

Martha boiled the kettle and filled a bucket of lukewarm water. I retrieved some arm-length gloves, a stomach tube, a funnel and lubricant from the car. Then under the vet's recommendation, we once again found ourselves entering the elephant enclosure, this time with Martha, to capture the infant elephant for one last time.

In the horse, I'd pass a nasogastric tube up the nose and down into the stomach to deliver an oral solution of rehydrating electrolyte fluid therapy. But the rather lengthy and hypermobile trunk of an elephant makes this approach impossible, so instead, the tube was coated with jelly lubricant and passed up his backside. Moments later, a funnel was attached to the outside end of the tube, Martha elevated it to her head height and the water steadily syphoned into the elephant's colon, very similar to how you might top up the screenwash in your car.

I placed my hand into his mouth and felt his tongue circle my fist. 'He's still got a good suckle reflex,' I quietly informed Martha. She raised her eyebrows with a judicious optimism.

'What about some jam?' I said, as I continued to gather my equipment back into the examination box and packed away the tube and funnel. 'To encourage a weak foal to suckle, I've seen some vets coat the mare's teat with strawberry jam.' Martha looked at me as though I had finally lost the plot. 'I don't know how feasible it is, or whether elephants like jam, but I guess you could try it.' I nodded over to the mother elephant who had watched us yet again interfere with her calf and let out two more trumpet blows to warn us of her discontent.

And, having delivered my old wives' tale of witchcraft and wizardry, I left them to it. As I travelled back to the practice, I kept wondering whether my efforts would make any difference at all to the overall outlook for the young elephant calf and prayed there would be no delays on any inbound flights that afternoon.

Monday morning soon arrived and I walked into work to find the team sharing drunk disco photos from the wedding and discussing the lavish reception, the free-flowing wine and the horror of the two-day hangover they'd all returned home with. I hadn't heard back from the zoo or Martha over the remainder of the weekend. But as the days ticked by, my mind kept wandering back to the elephant calf and the most bizarre weekend of my veterinary career. Generally speaking, no news is good news with our patients. Safe in the knowledge that the zoo vet would have taken over, I knew there was little chance they would need to contact us again. Still, I was desperate to know how things had played out, for better or worse. And so, I decided to drop Martha an email. It took a few days, but eventually a reply came:

James,

You'll be pleased to hear the newborn elephant calf turned a corner and is now doing well. He had a plasma transfusion and is still on antibiotics. We have sent blood off to check for elephant endotheliotropic herpesvirus (EEHV), although this is more for completeness and we won't get the results back for another few weeks. Astrid, the zoo vet, is still not entirely sure what caused his neurological signs, but he looks set to make a good recovery. I have attached a quick video for you to see the transformation. I also thought you might like to know we have named him 'Lenny', short for 'Khi len' – meaning 'playful' as he is a joyous little character!

Thank you for your help.

Best,

Martha Van Heerden

P.S. He now loves strawberry jam!

CHAPTER 10

Rudy

(This chapter contains a description of severe animal cruelty and abuse that may be distressing.)

'Zrrrrr, zrrrrr, zrrrrr ... Beep, beep, beep ... Zrrrrr, zrrrr ...'

I reached over to the bedside table, grabbed the rectangular black plastic pager and hit the silence button. The familiar, inevitable bolt of 'fight or flight' anxiety zip-wired through every nerve fibre in my body – from my toes to the pit of my stomach, then to my fingertips and finally my eyelids, when immediately they sprang open and I was wide awake. It was 4.45 a.m.

There is no feeling quite like going from the mental 'relaxation' of being asleep to suddenly being fully awake, shocked into action to engage the exhausted grey matter and enable an immediate conversation with a pet owner to reassure, diagnose and offer advice without sounding like a half-tranquillized buffoon. I would, at best, only catnap through the nights when on call. And it being my full duty weekend, I'd be lucky if I managed anything more than a few hours over the standard eighty-two-hour shift.*

I placed the silenced pager on my bedside table and pulled the covers back, knowing more was to come. And right on cue came the inevitable '*der, der, der, derrrr . . . der, der, der*' of my work Nokia mobile phone. I had placed the phone a distance away from the pager, and out of arm's reach. A tactical move to curb my 'snooze button' tendencies, as I could never quite trust my semi-conscious brain not to silence the disturbance and allow me to fall back to sleep.

I read the charcoal-grey pixellated letters form into words as they flashed across the pager display. 'Horse with colic. Reggie. Will Benson, Lower Hagg Farm. Pls call first.' A horse with colic was perhaps the most common reason for being called out of hours. Colic is essentially the horsey equivalent to a human with indigestion, or perhaps trapped wind, except, left untreated, it can quickly progress from being something mild to something fatal. So perhaps 'indigestion' is not a fair analogy at all. In fact, colic is probably one of the most common causes of death in horses, although these days the stats and prognoses for a favourable outcome are far better. So it's more like compounding all the indigestion you've ever

---

* To give an insight into my working hours as a junior vet at that time, the on-call shift was Friday evening to Monday morning. But, as I worked full days on the Friday and Monday, the actual workable shift without a break was from 8.30 a.m. Friday morning until 6.30 p.m. Monday evening. We would usually work Monday to Friday, and then Friday to Monday on call into the new week, then from Monday to Thursday with the following Friday off. So that's eleven days of work, which we were scheduled to do every fifth week on the rota.

had in your life and rolling it up into one supersized mega bout of your stomach doing literal somersaults, twisting and turning on itself.

Colic in all its forms is always a worry for any horse owner, and is always taken seriously by vets. The 'morning colic' is of particular concern, though, as no one can say for sure at what time during the night the symptoms first began and it is therefore hard to know how far along a sliding scale the horse is towards developing life-threatening toxic physiological changes.

After refusing his morning breakfast, an educated guess suggested that Reggie was heading into a nasty bout. I dialled the telephone number. An alert, busy young man's voice answered. 'Hiya, yep, you'll have to come straight out, please. He's off his hay, pawing his front leg and trying to lie down.* I've got a head collar on him and we're just walking gently round the yard.'

Without doubt, Reggie needed to be seen. I pulled on my navy polo shirt and my stone chinos (the left knee of which was stained with a dried 'watermark', having being saturated by kneeling in the juicy straw bedding of a gelding whose fetlock had needed a dressing change about six hours before Reggie's owner had called). I pulled on my sturdy boots with their fairly distinct sweet ammonia 'horsey' smell, got in the car and set off in the dark to locate my next patient.

I pulled up to the old, cobbled farm drive. Reggie was owned by a guy in his late thirties. He wore a baseball cap, keeping his dark chestnut-brown hair swept back, and he had a kind, gentle way about him. But he was absolutely no

---

* These are classic colic symptoms.

pushover. We had crossed paths a few times and I knew he was an experienced horseman. I had met Reggie as one of my first patients after joining the practice when I was called to dig a pocket of pus out from his front right hoof. His owner had more or less guided me to exactly where he had predicted the abscess to be, and sure enough, with the confirmation of the hoof testers, he was absolutely on the mark. This was an owner who knew his horse well.

It was just gone 5 a.m. and in late autumn, the sun wouldn't rise for another few hours. I swung the vehicle through the farm gates and into the cobbled yard, then dropped my full beam. Between my dipped headlights and the single halogen bulb attached over Reggie's stable door, there was just enough light to illuminate a section of the farmyard. Through the shadows, I could just make out the profile of the huge seventeen-hand gelding as he walked towards my car, with a rope leading from the underside of his chin to the worried hand of his owner, Will.

He looked at least twice his height, yet I had no doubt Will had complete control of him. I killed the engine but left the headlights on. As I stepped out from the car, I heard the familiar voice from the telephone. As they continued to walk slowly towards me, Reggie suddenly stopped and threw his head up high before dropping his nose to the ground, reaching forwards with a front hoof and flaring his nostrils with each exhale, blowing the small shards of straw and debris from the cracks between the cobbles. He rubbed the bridge of his nose against the front wall of his foreleg.

'No, no, no, no!' Will said, as he tightened up the lead rope to pull his head back into a more neutral position. But before he could, Reggie swung his head violently to the right, then shook his head which pulled Will round and almost toppled him onto the cobbles. 'REGGIE!' he called, the tone of a shocked and worried owner. It was a subconscious reaction, more out of surprise that Reggie would be so disregarding of Will's presence, pulling him about so abruptly. A horse's head alone equates to around 10 per cent of their total body weight, and so the vast, dense musculature running along the neck is no match for any human to compete against. But to throw his strength around like that was totally out of character for such a gentle, kind-natured horse. Without any doubt, he was trying to tell us that he was in pain.

We exchanged greetings. I stroked the palm of my hand along Reggie's neck. This was the first time Reggie had suffered with a bout of colic and Will was fully aware of the gravitas and uncertainty that colic can bring. The first deciding factor of assessing a horse with colic is the pulse rate. I took the stethoscope from around my neck and placed the drum against his chest wall. I isolated the sound to the thud of the heart – rhythmic, regular, and only moderately elevated. Good news. Hopefully.

I continued my exam. Reggie's gum colour was a pale salmon-pink – also a good sign. His temperature was normal too. I manoeuvred my stethoscope across the quadrants of his abdomen and listened to his gut sounds. It is quite normal to hear a whole plethora of groans, croaks and whooshing sounds, like water being flushed down the toilet. When these sounds are absent, the worry is there may be a blockage. But in Reggie's case, it was like placing a microphone and recording the sounds from a local launderette – swirling, whooshing, gurgling and burping sounds reverberated across all four sections of his abdomen.

I explained to Will that this seemed most likely to be a spasmodic colic, the kind that would hopefully respond well to medical management. I drew a number of liquid medications from glass bottles in the boot of my car and plunged a thick-gauged needle into the drain-pipe jugular vein that ran up the left side of Reggie's neck. I allowed some blood to run through the needle – to ensure it was a gentle trickle and not the pulsating jet of an artery. As the warm blood trickled over my skin, I kept the needle in place with my right hand and connected each syringe in turn, slowly flooding his bloodstream with soothing painkillers and anti-spasmodic medications to relive the abdominal cramping. We discussed the signs to watch for, I packed my car and left Reggie and Will to it.

A few hours later, a second text arrived to my phone saying, 'Reggie so much better, thank you. Should be fine from here, will only call again if worried. Cheers, Will.' It was the update I had hoped for.

With time, I began to hone my clinical skills and develop a 'veterinary gut instinct'. I learnt to read my animal patient's behaviour, pick up on their symptoms, categorise the severity and decide whether they were improving or deteriorating, critical or stable and whether they carried a good, fair, poor or grave prognosis. No two days were ever the same, but there were often similarities that I started to draw across different situations to help me build up a bank of experiences – a little black book of possible, or probable, or unrelated outcomes to reflect and draw upon. As I look back now with hindsight, my 'gut instinct' at the time was probably all part of the process of me transitioning from an inexperienced to an experienced vet. Yet, no matter how far along I continue in my career, there are a handful of situations that still haunt me to this day. Situations where my gut instinct or experience offered little reassurance; those few exceptional cases that I could never have prepared for. The cases that lie beyond the scope of the textbooks, beyond the remit of day-to-day vetting, and instead opened my eyes to the darkest corners of society.

I had felt the pager buzz against my waist, attached to the belt of my trousers. Five new text messages from worried horse owners. This was not hugely unusual for a Sunday morning, the calls normally arrived early doors. Five a.m. starts are pretty standard for horse owners, and weekends were no exception. Usually, it was around these 'checkpoint' times – feeding, grooming, turning out – that problems were spotted and the vet would be called.

I worked out the geography of each call to formulate a route and gave an expected arrival time to each. Five horses may not sound a lot, but more could call at any time. And with over five hundred horses on the books, spread over a fifty-mile radius, and only me on call representing a five-vet team, it was certainly enough to be getting on with.

As dawn broke and I pulled up to each yard, the horses presented themselves with a variety of ailments. More colicking ponies, limping legs and snotty noses. And still the pager continued to vibrate.

'Horse coughing two days. Pls call for advice.'

'Limping near fore, can't walk. Pls call on Mrs mob.'

'Wound on leg. Just happened. Poss kicked in field. Call urgent.'

By mid-afternoon the calls became fewer and further between. I managed to get home, made a cup of tea, and hoped the laundered polo shirt and second set of chinos I had left on the lukewarm radiators were dry enough to exchange for the heavily soiled uniform I'd worn for thirty-six hours straight. I grabbed the beige trousers in the palm of my hand and repeatedly squeezed the hem and waistband to assess whether they were dry enough to wear – weighing up whether to stay smelling like an equine lavatory for a little longer or switch trousers and risk putting up with a slightly humid inner thigh as I volunteered myself as a human clothes horse.

While I pontificated, I heard the pager buzz once more. I left the trousers draped over the sofa and seized an opportunity to slurp a decent gulp of tea. As I stood with the warm mug of tea in one hand, I read as the letters traversed along the thin rectangular screen. Frustrated to know I'd be back on the road within minutes, I only offered it half my attention, expecting to read about another colic, or another lame horse, or another owner trying to book in an 'emergency' vaccination, being the weekend and hoping I might be passing by. I slurped the tea, and over the rim of the mug, I caught a glimpse of only two words: 'horse' and 'fire'.

Surely a typo. The remote answering service was there to act as a bit of a 'buffer', to remind the public this was an emergency service and not a direct 24/7 line to a vet for general enquires. The calls were initially received by a call centre, the message would then be transcribed to the duty vet in a neat, succinct package on the pager and a more detailed version texted to the work mobile phone. As such, it wasn't *that* unusual to get a few anomalies. 'Owner to pick up their boot? Outside practice now', for example, meant an owner had arrived to collect some pain relief, in the form of phenylbutazone, often shortened to the slang term 'bute' and had absolutely nothing to do with equine or human footwear.

I picked up the phone to see if I might be able to glean any further insight from the unabridged version of the message. I opened the home screen, tapped onto the text message and read it in full. This was no typo.

'HORSE ON FIRE. URGENT. PLS CALL ON MOB IMMEDIATELY.'

What? I immediately dialled the telephone number attached. After only one ring, a croaky female voice answered. ''Ello?' she said.

'Hi, it's James calling from the vet's—' but before I could finish my usual patter of enquiry into how I could help, the voice cut in.

'Oh my God, he's been set on fire! You need to come now.' Her voice was shaky, clearly in shock. 'Please just help me!' Her voice broke. The phone fell silent as she was unable to speak through her tears. I could hear a group of distanced voices through the handset.

'Hello?' I shouted through the phone. 'Hello? Can you hear me?'

It is not unusual for owners in a state of shock to drop the phone or lower it away from their ears. Suddenly, her voice returned. 'Yeah, I'm here. Can you come?'

'Yes. Is everyone safe? Have you phoned the fire brigade?' I asked, imagining a stable block or barn alight.

'What? No, no, yeah, everyone's fine,' she said, confused. 'Just please come!' I could hear crying in the background, a distressed high-pitched shrieking cry that sounded like a teenage girl in horror.

I left the tea on the kitchen table, grabbed my keys and ran to the car. I didn't recognise the address – they weren't registered clients of ours. So I tapped the postcode into Google

Maps – the flag dropped onto the edge of what looked like a heavily residential area. It made no sense. Horses are kept in all sort of places: rented paddocks, shared livery yards, million-pound mansions, race yards, but never before had I been called to somewhere as built up as this. Google told me I was about thirty-five minutes' drive away. I sped down our quiet lane and onto the main A-road, shouting profanities over the top of my steering wheel, as I looked up at the red bulb of the traffic light. Sitting stationary, I tried to focus my mind on all the potential consequences, and importantly, the emergency triage of burn wounds. As the traffic light held me still further, the minutes felt like hours.

The blue line of the Google map eventually showed the chequered flag, indicating I had reached my destination. The tarmac road was lined with beige-coloured, rendered houses. There was smashed glass on the pavement, and a St George flag suspended in front of the white net curtain of an upstairs window with a dog barking at the door. I pulled over slowly. A man in his late twenties was standing against the fence panel of one of the houses. He had pale skin and dark circles around both his eyes, exaggerated by the shade of the baseball cap protruding over his brow. He took a drag of the cigarette he had clasped between his thumb and forefinger that he cupped with the palm of his hand. He stared as I climbed out from the car, nodding at me without breaking his expression.

'I'm looking for someone called Carrie?' I called over to him.

He turned his head and nodded in the direction of the street. 'Last house on the right,' he said, pointing with the hand that held the cigarette. Then he looked the other way and took another toke on his cigarette before he rolled his tongue around his mouth and spat a ball of phlegm onto the ground.

I got back in the car and continued to snake along the street. A young girl was stood on the roadside curb. Her head was bowed. Her locks of bleached-blonde curls formed a curtain around the mobile phone she was staring down at in her hands. She had a pair of wellington boots on, short denim shorts and a tight black T-shirt with the word 'Miami' written in block capitals, printed across the front. Her legs were crossed, as though she had been waiting there a long time, expecting someone to arrive. That someone was likely me.

'Hi, are you Carrie?' I asked.

'No. Are you the vet?' she asked back.

'I am, yeah.'

'Come through 'ere.'

I grabbed my stethoscope and surreptitiously tucked the case of veterinary drugs under a large coat on the back seat, and then covered it with some less inviting, uninteresting veterinary paraphernalia. I followed her through an alleyway between two houses. The fence boundary was littered with Coke cans, smashed bottles and used yellow polystyrene food containers that looked as though they would have once contained a doner kebab from the row of takeaway shops I passed on the precinct at the end of the road. We trampled further along the alleyway and I caught the faint sound of voices. As we neared, the alleyway opened up into a stretch of generic grassy scrubland, bordered by houses, and in the centre was a vast electricity pylon. The triangular metal frame of the pylon erupted from the ground like a man-made industrial volcano. Various suspended cables towered above us and a main A-road concrete flyover crossed the farthest boundary channelling the many vehicles that shot past. The Sunday traffic was light, but the noise of the occasional passing lorry still rumbled loudly down the valley as it shuddered past. Some wire fencing, patched up in places, provided the boundary to create a horse's paddock, and in the distance a simple field shelter offered some respite from the elements.

The girl guided me over to a group of people, most of whom looked a similar age to her. They all stood in a huddle staring at their mobile phones – frantically tapping and showing each other their screens. One girl at the centre of the group looked particularly overwhelmed and distraught. Her eyes were brick red; black mascara on her eyelashes had leached down her face, creating rivers of black tarry tears across both her cheeks. She had her head pressed against the chest of her friend, who cradled her in her arms as she sobbed. As we approached, an older lady stepped forwards from the group. Her eyes were also bloodshot and her fingernails tapped furiously on the screen of her mobile phone. She was upset. But what had started as tears of sadness had soon melted into anger.

'Hi,' I said. 'I'm the vet, I think we spoke on the phone.'

'Hiya, yeah, I'm Carrie. I'm sorry, I'm just really pissed off at the . . .' Her breath caught short, she stopped talking and inhaled deeply, and as she filled her lungs fresh tears began to well in her eyes. 'I'm gonna fuckin' kill whoever's done this, I swear.' She turned and looked away from me, curling both her forefingers and placed them against her lower eyelids in an attempt to stem the overflowing tears of emotions. She sniffed to clear the watery liquid running from her eyes and down her nose. Then continued: 'He's over here. You'd better come and 'av a look at him.'

Carrie led me past the group of teenage girls and her daughter, still in the arms of her friend's comforting embrace. The daughter managed to mouth the word 'hi' before she turned her head back into her friend's chest and broke into a continued, agonising sob. It was her horse, her first horse, whom she loved dearly and had named Rudy.

Another woman was holding on to the lead rein and in front of us stood a hairy, gentle-faced horse. Rudy was a cob; sturdy, with stout stumpy legs and markings that made him look like a Friesian cow, or a dalmatian dog – with big splodges of black and white all over his body and down his legs. He would perhaps be deemed as 'nothing special' according to the fairly judgemental horsey world, but I could sense by their reaction that, despite their simple set-up, he was adored by his owner and meant the world to them.

As we walked towards Rudy, he clocked us approaching, threw his head up then started to tiptoe his four feet on the spot before finally he took two large steps back. A classic fear response. He was afraid of me.

'OK, OK. Good boy, it's OK.' I spoke quietly, but on recognising that my very presence was making him increasingly nervous, I stopped still and remained silent.

He was clearly apprehensive and needed some time to become accustomed, so I waited – and began to take in as much information as I could from a distance. Yet even though I was just a few feet away, there wasn't anything I could immediately spot. As I stood in front of him, his face, neck and shoulders all looked normal. There was no blood, he wasn't struggling for breath and from the few strides he had just taken, I could see he wasn't overtly lame. He looked scared, but on the whole he seemed OK. I turned back to Carrie. 'So what's actually happened then?'

'You'll see but you'll 'ave to come round the side,' she said, manoeuvring herself round from his head to the flank of his body. But as she did so, Rudy also spun on the spot at the same pace, reluctant to allow any of us out of his direct eyeline. 'There! Did you see?'

The truth is, I couldn't see anything. Every time Carrie had stepped to the side, Rudy kept up, which meant from where I was standing, I could only see his front profile. 'All right, let me take a look?'

Carrie stood back. She continued to wipe her eyes and cheeks with a tissue, then waved it impatiently in the air to silence a shout from the group of teenagers eager to know what was being said.

I moved into place and replicated her steps. And with each large sidestep stride I took, Rudy circled with me, as predicted – hiding his back end and keeping me in his direct line of vision. This time, though, I did manage to clock the horror of what had happened. 'Bloody hell!' I muttered under my breath.

Only the briefest glimpse of the hair on Rudy's rump, normally a thick coat of off-white/grey hair, told me everything I needed to know. The only way I can describe it would be to imagine someone climbing a ladder and pouring a can of paint down the back of this poor animal. Although for Rudy, instead of paint, it had been a can of petrol. Doused in fuel. And then set alight. The flame had burnt through his coat in seconds and then to the skin beneath, which had in turn melted into a scorched and blistered black patch of permanent scarring. Like flesh left too long on an unmanned barbecue, the charred skin on his rump demonstrated where the petrol had initially pooled, then where it had splashed and dribbled down his hind legs. And where the accelerant had dripped, the dancing flames had soon leapt and followed in close pursuit. A splash pattern of unimaginable pain. The unmistakable smell of burnt hair wafted as Rudy continued to spin on the spot, almost purposefully, I imagined, through the cooling autumn air.

'What the hell?' I turned and looked to Carrie. 'I've never seen anything like it!'

Normally, I'd never confess this in front of a client – an immediate admission of inexperience. But I had *never* seen anything like it. My own shock and gut reaction had put the impulsive words straight into my mouth.

'You 'aven't seen the worst yet,' Carrie replied. She lifted her phone, turned the handset on its side and tilted it slightly towards my direction.

There's something quite intrusive about looking at another person's phone, so I glanced away and continued my assessment of Rudy. But I could hear the tapping of her nails against the screen.

'Here, look!'

I knelt slightly and cupped my hand over the screen to shade it from the dull, grey daylight sky. Though buffering and still downloading, I immediately recognised the white triangle within a red rectangle as YouTube. After a few seconds, a shaky, pixellated video started to play. A group of young voices shouted in the background, then the blurred yet characteristic black and white markings of a horse came into view. It was Rudy, leaning his face forwards over a barbed-wire fence. His face looked relaxed, friendly, hopeful even, perhaps for a polo mint or a surprise apple revealed from someone's pocket. The video was jumpy, it panned the ground, then to someone's feet, then up to a coat pocket, across to Rudy, then back to the ground.

'Do it, g'wan!' A male voice.

With the phone camera still angled to the ground, a sloshing sound could be heard.

'Yeah, g'wan now! Yeah, I'm filmin', yeah.' The same creaky, broken voice of a teenage boy.

There was shouting, maybe four or five different voices. High-pitched, erratic teenage squeals from girls and the nervous profanities from boys, all egging someone into action. Then the camera lifted. Rudy came back into view, first his neck lifted, his face rose out of shot, then he turned, quickly, and ran. He galloped, quickly out of view, beyond the capabilities of the early phone camera. But as he sped away, a ball of white light followed him. The light had overexposed on the screen and totally bleached out any definition of what was really happening. Although looking at the burns on his skin, it was quite clear exactly what had happened. Rudy was on fire. To the laughs, the torments and the hyper-stimulated voices of a group of teenagers. They swore, laughed, jeered and relished in every single second of the adrenaline-fuelled rush they had created for themselves.

Carrie dropped the phone to her waist and stared at me. 'Can you believe it?' she asked quietly. *How could anyone believe it?* 'Bastards filmed it. Then sent a link to my daughter. It's what they're all watching now.' She nodded over to the group of crying teenage girls. 'Tormenting herself, she thinks it's her fault!' Carrie continued. 'I'll fucking kill 'em,' she finished with, as new tears pooled along her lower eyelids, overflowed, then trickled down both her cheeks one after the other. She wiped them away, this time aggressively, using the palm of her hands, as she switched from maternal worry for her daughter's welfare to an unquenched thirst for revenge on each and every one of the perpetrators of the crime that had inflicted such trauma on her family, of which Rudy was clearly a treasured member.

What was I going to do? How do you treat the extensive petrol burns of an animal's skin? This was beyond the veterinary textbooks, no lecture notes to refer back to, no experienced colleague to draw on. *Nobody* had ever seen anything like this. Furthermore, there is no NHS for pets. That is a fact. I knew that the burns in front of me were only the very tip of the iceberg for what was to follow. Rudy needed to be admitted to the equine hospital. He would need twenty-four-hour care. Burn wounds often worsen before they improve. I knew there was a distinct and very real risk that the skin across his entire back end was likely to slough. The full extent of how much damage had been done would not reveal itself for many days to come. Slow, steady, supportive care was needed. Multiple wound dressings with daily, repeat sedations to apply them. Blood tests to continually assess for protein loss, and to ensure Rudy didn't fall into organ failure as the burnt skin exerted its effect upon Rudy's entire physiology. Intravenous antibiotic injections, bandages, painkilling injections. The list went on. Knowing the pricing structure of the practice (which employed vets, such as myself, have no say in) and the fact Rudy would need at least four weeks of continual care, I knew his care would easily run into many thousands of pounds. And this is very difficult to admit, but my immediate reaction to this particular situation was to question whether the cost may prohibit his treatment, and if so, whether I may need to consider humanely putting Rudy to sleep.

I truly struggle with this aspect of veterinary medicine. Not the fact that there is a bill, or that we charge for our services. What I find the hardest is that the employed vet, the GP vet, is usually the one on the ground, at the coalface, whose shoulders it lands on to absorb the grief, upset, verbal abuse and emotional blackmail when it comes to the cost of veterinary medicine. I don't set the fees or take a bonus cut of my turnover; my salary stays fixed regardless of my work. But still, it's the employed vet that gets subjected to phrases such as 'You are supposed to care.' 'Daylight robbery.' 'Just a licence to print money.' I've heard it all. This is the side of veterinary medicine that doesn't often get spoken about in the media. It's more romantic to paint a picture whereby the vet plays the hero, the animal guru who steps in and heals all. But the reality is, there is always a cost involved somewhere. And that cost can be the difference between whether an animal receives care, and a chance for survival, or not. But euthanasia is not a dirty word or an admission of failure. Every situation is unique. I don't believe it is morally right to do a 'half job' and leave an animal to suffer. Something you learn as a vet is that through hindsight, you can gain the benefit of foresight. You can have an appreciation of what is to follow and what is around the corner. The burns on Rudy were excruciatingly painful and a *significant* risk to his life. Burying our heads in the sand or opting for a 'let's just wait and see' approach would have been handing Rudy a slow, painful death sentence. It was the conversation I was dreading.

'I'm going to have to be really frank with you, Carrie,' I said, as I tried to explain the complexities and potential cost of treatment. I can imagine it seems insensitive that I brought up cost when there is an owner who is in such distress, and a horse that has suffered through no fault of its own. But this is the reality of being an employee, a front-line vet.

'Just do whatever you need,' she said.

Words which should, of course, sound comforting. But words are easily spoken. She wasn't a registered client, I had no history on Carrie or her financial background and I knew I would be hauled in front of the boss for agreeing to treatment to an unregistered client without payment upfront.

'OK, but we're likely to be talking about several thousands of pounds here.'

'Yeah, it's OK, just do it,' she said. 'He's got full insurance and no exclusions apart from lameness as he had a foot abscess two years ago.'

The words I had so desperately longed to hear. The fact she had invested in a thorough insurance policy meant Rudy had just been thrown a lifeline, a hope for survival.

Rudy was transported to the hospital. Carrie and her daughter visited daily. A potent cocktail of opiate pain relief mixed with saline, his fluid therapy trickled through the cannula plugged into his jugular vein day and night. The burnt 'splash' wound on his back end did, as predicted, spread. Daily measurements showed the full extent of trauma. Like lava, the burn wound slowly crept further and further each day, the edges of his skin burnt bright red as the charred top layer of epidermis peeled away. A burn cream made from colloidal silver was applied twice a day, antiseptic, soothing, healing. Tub after tub, tube after tube, to maintain a thick barrier layer of ointment across the skin surface. By day, the nursing team cleaned and dressed his wounds, administered his medication and kept him fed, watered and able to rest in a clean bed. And, through many hands and collective effort, he started to make a slow recovery.

What I remember the most about Rudy, aside from the horrific physical abuse, is the emotional trauma he had suffered at the hands of human beings. His experience of people up to that point had made him into a confident, loving, trusting companion, comfortable in the company of others. Within seconds that bond had been broken. His eyes, as I stood in the field and attempted to examine his back, were filled with such distrust. His head held high, the whites of his eyes glared at me so brightly as he skipped about on all four feet. Any closer and he was ready to rear. His survival instincts had been triggered and from that moment on he saw all unfamiliar humans as a potential threat.

Every day, I took food. I took treats. I took peace offerings. Yet every time I walked close, he backed off. Not from the other vets or the nurses; with time they could enter the stable without him moving a muscle. But he linked me to his pain in that field. And so the kindest thing I could do was not to challenge him. I stepped back from his primary care – the trauma was perhaps too much for both of us to bear – but I kept taking him food, hoping to rebuild some of the trust. And gradually, after many weeks, there was some progress. As the days passed, his wounds healed and the trust slowly grew. He still kept all four feet firmly planted on the spot in my presence, but eventually he would cautiously stretch his neck forwards, like a giraffe reaching for the furthest branch of a tree, as he gently nuzzled a carrot from my outstretched hand with his big floppy lips.

After almost five weeks, Rudy was eventually discharged from the hospital and allowed to continue his treatment at home. Carrie wrapped a head collar over his nose and round his thick neck and he walked comfortably and calmly towards the horse box. As he did, he looked round one last time, and there was the face I will for ever remember. Even after all he had been through, both the physical and mental trauma, all Rudy really wanted was to be reunited with the family he loved, the humans he trusted, and to go home. His scars were not his weakness, but a reminder of his strength, resilience and determination. Of course, I was delighted to see him make a full recovery and even more to hear of a successful prosecution.

A lot of time has passed since I got the call-out to help Rudy, but I still think of him often. His story is perhaps one of the most horrific acts I have ever witnessed. Sadly, though, after fifteen years as a vet, he is not the only animal I have seen suffer at the hands of humans. But he was the first. And it is only now I can look back and recognise how these incredibly intense and emotionally traumatic experiences have likely affected my own mental health. At the time I bottled it up. And I know there will be many others in this industry, under the same self-induced pressure to remain 'ever professional', who have done the same.

It was one thing to witness something so horrific, but then to also feel the weight of responsibility to make it all better – his treatment, his rehabilitation, his trust. All eyes were on Rudy, and therefore all eyes were on me. Would he pull through? Would he recover? I felt an immense pressure on my shoulders to make all this right. The truth is, of course, it wasn't all on my shoulders. The incredible veterinary team rallied, his care became a real practice-wide effort. But to revisit his trauma on a daily basis was still very heavy-going. I know now that I should have spoken up about how much it affected me. But even now I wonder whether I would have accepted support or help, even if it had been offered to me. The guilt of leaving my colleagues short, asking them to pick up extra work to allow me to take a break, or simply accepting that I was the one who needed help, would have left me feeling weak – the weakest link in a chain of toughened, competitive vets. In my mind, they could all cope, so why couldn't I?

There are distressing statistics around the mental health and suicide rates of vets and veterinary nurses. According to a published study, vets are three to four times more likely to die by suicide than the general population.* The huge question remains 'why?' Obviously I can only speak to my personal experience on this point. For me, it was not a causative relationship; veterinary medicine did not *cause* me to spiral – and I think it is important for the profession to differentiate between a situation that is caused by the job and one that is exacerbated by it. I firmly believe that my having poor mental health was not an inevitable consequence of working as a vet. Having said that, there were certain aspects of my working life as a vet that undoubtedly contributed to it. At a time in my life when I was already going through a difficult period, the intensely stressful conversations and sometimes incredibly traumatic experiences that come with being a vet

---

* Vetlife.org.uk (Platt et al. 2010).

didn't help my already dwindling sense of being able to cope. When I look back now it is clear to me that the ethical and moral dilemmas that come with the job, as well as the clinical decision-making involved with providing veterinary health-care on a daily basis, and the roller coaster of upset or joy that both brought, had started to create a form of traumatic stress within me. For those working in healthcare, this is a specific form of burnout known as 'compassion fatigue'. *

It was never a case of losing compassion for the animals under my care – in fact, it was the animals that kept me going a lot of the time. But opening my heart and mind to the animals and owners I saw on a daily basis was taking its toll on my own health. If empathy was a currency, then I was rapidly heading towards bankruptcy. I had offered so much of myself to veterinary medicine. In caring for my patients, I had exhausted all my reserves and had subconsciously stopped caring for myself.

It had started to cause arguments at home, I had started to make unhealthy choices and I had even started to question whether it was time for me to hang up my childhood dream and take a different career path altogether. Nearly every day I would ask myself whether this really was the best job in the world or whether I'd been missold a dream that was

---

* According to VetLife, a charity that provides support to members of the UK veterinary community and their families who have emotional, health or financial concerns and seeks ways to prevent such situations in the future, vets 'commonly attribute their psychological distress to these problems at work: work intensity (pace and volume); duration of working hours and its associated effects on personal lives; feeling undervalued by senior staff and/or management; performance anxiety – particularly if recently qualified'.

slowly turning into a nightmare. Tragically, by this point in my career, I had also lost a close colleague to suicide. I still find it hard to talk about. It is not my story to tell in any sort of detail – and I'm certainly not trying to conflate or compare the two experiences here – but having experienced first-hand all the rippling emotions that another person's suicide can bring, those of sadness, guilt, anger and inward concern for my own mental health, I think it is actually so very important that we do start talking about this. And I firmly believe those conversations have to start from within the profession.

No job is ever perfect, but for me it went a step further. I was teetering on the edge of falling out of love with veterinary medicine altogether. I had fallen into a cycle of blaming all my frustrations in life on it and came so very close to jacking it all in – a profession I had once loved, my passion, my vocation, something I had worked so hard at to get to where I was.

It hurts to write this now, as I'm in such a different place and my feelings towards veterinary are so much more positive. With hindsight, though, if I could go back, this was the time when I ought to have overcome the stigma and sought professional help. But I didn't. And I'm sure I am not alone in that.

Within the vast majority of veterinary practices, there is still no proper opportunity for staff to decompress, no easy access to regular peer support or the opportunity to safely and routinely talk with a mental health professional trained specifically in helping members of the veterinary profession. There are some fantastic, fully confidential charities,* but

---

* Please see the resources section at the end of the book for charities and organisations that can help.

these rely either on an individual vet being brave enough and self-aware enough to reach out, or on a strong enough support system being in place within the practice to encourage this. To anyone reading this who feels this way, whether working in the veterinary industry or not, I want to say now – loud and clear – that asking for and accepting help is absolutely never anything to be ashamed of. I wish I had known that back then.

CHAPTER 11

Alice

'C'mon,' the owner said to her slightly bored-looking dog being dragged along three paces behind as she burst through the practice doors. She walked straight up to the reception desk and then, instead of making eye contact, looked down at her watch and said, 'Err, it's Alice. She's here for a booster.'

It was 8.46 a.m. Alice's owner was dressed in a black pencil skirt, a white blouse and a black blazer. She was very much in a hurry and she felt the need for others to know. She had a badge on her lapel that read 'Jackie Richardson – Consultant Solicitor', next to the logo of a legal firm. A nest of wild, curly, blonde hair was paired with her maroon-painted fingernails and there was a faint scent of nicotine about her that her morning spritz of honey-ish perfume was failing to disguise. 'I'm in a bit of a rush,' she rudely instructed.

'Yep, that's OK, just take a seat,' the receptionist said. 'You are quite early but I'll go and see if I've got a vet free.'

The consult room door that led to the reception area had been left partly open, so I overheard the exchange of words

202

while I was sitting at my computer, scrolling and clicking my way through some lab reports and a list of unread internal emails.

Please note, Clindafloxacillin is out of stock until further notice. Delete.

A reminder: Can all staff please park on the road and not take a space in the car park. Delete.

THE KITCHEN IS DISGUSTING. Please can we ALL do our own washing-up – including cleaning the microwave if you're making soup! Delete.

My growing indignation was broken only by the squeak of the receptionist's chair as she stood to come and ask how I might feel about picking up an early consult. Take one for the team, as they say. I was one step ahead, though. I'd already clocked that if I could rattle through the booster, Jackie Richardson might be happy at my super-efficient approach to veterinary medicine and I'd be able to steal a second brew before the onslaught of the back-to-back consults set to fill my morning. I stood up from my desk, walked into reception, acknowledged our receptionist with a silent nod as if to say, 'I'm already on it!', then called Alice through.

Alice was a German shepherd crossed with a Border collie, two breeds with notoriously fast reactions. But Alice had proven all stereotypes wrong. She was pretty chilled or, maybe I should say, 'unreactive'. She didn't particularly mind being checked over. I'd seen her for the previous year's booster and made a point to record on her notes that she was 'very well-behaved for the examination' as code to any future colleagues that may notice her breed combination and need a little reassurance on which way her temperament had swayed.

It is not about pre-judging any particular breed, but certain breed personality traits do manifest when faced with challenging situations. A trip to the vet's is stressful for most dogs. It is an onslaught on all their senses – the smells, the sounds, lots of humans and lots of other animals, all in close proximity. Some animals may be in pain, others may not be used to company, some may want to play, others will bark, and some will freeze in fear. A visit to the vet's must be hugely triggering for most animals. While a springer spaniel may walk into the consulting room and typically roll onto their back, present their belly, sweep their tail side to side and possibly even pass urine, a Border collie would more characteristically start with lots of 'snuggle behaviour', get as close to me as possible, freeze, then watch me from the corner of their eye, sometimes with a very low grumble. Then, often, they will immediately resume the snuggle behaviour in an attempt to befriend the 'thing' that they perceived as a threat (i.e. me!). A cockerpoo might be conflicted between wanting to approach and engage but then finds the whole concept too overwhelming and so chooses instead to run behind the legs of their owner. And then there is the Labrador that comes in and immediately sits patiently by the owner's feet, freezes and trembles. ALL these dogs are showing signs that they are anxious about being at the vet's, they just express it in different ways.

It is not about pitching breeds against each other as being 'friendly' or 'dangerous' – breed shaming or compiling a list of so-called 'dangerous dogs' in law, based purely on their looks, to me (and many others) is completely farcical. And has been proven ineffective at reducing the heartbreaking statistics around dog bites and dog-related fatalities. In fifteen years, I've only *properly* been bitten once by a dog in my consulting room. Normally I'd say I am pretty adept at picking up a dog's body language, but this time the response came from nowhere. I say that now, but of course, if I reflect on it honestly, I had probably asked too much of him and my expectations for him to cooperate had stretched one step too far. The dog launched, I shielded myself with my left arm, the dog's teeth punctured the base of my thumb (the soft part of your hand that looks a bit like a chicken drumstick) and as I leapt backwards, he launched again and punctured my chin. Even then, I didn't blame the dog. He was responding to the situation he was in and I misread his body language. I did, however, shudder at the response of his owner who shrugged his shoulders and just said, 'Yeah, well, dogs bite, innit.' It has nothing to do with the breed of the dog.

As vets, we often have to do our best in a short space of time by making the most of various tactics to reduce a dog's anxiety while at the vet's: positive distraction techniques, for example, with treats or toys; recommending medication or referral to a clinical animal behaviourist. A muzzle, though, is often the only safe way to ensure all veterinary staff are kept safe and should not itself be stigmatised or taken offence at.*

---

* I think all dogs would benefit from being trained to wear a muzzle, not as a response to their behaviour but as a proactive, preventative tool should the situation arise where a vet (or owner) deems that a muzzle is required. If we all trained our dogs to happily put their nose into a muzzle for a piece of food in the calm home environment, the muzzle itself does not get linked to a negative experience and it wouldn't then cause extra stress if one was required. Most dogs can easily learn to accept wearing a muzzle like they do a collar. It is

Alice, though, stayed completely still; she didn't bark, she didn't wag her tail, she didn't even take any treats – she was, to all intents and purposes, 'pretty chilled'. Either chilled, or perhaps a little 'shut down'.

'Is she normally like this?' I asked inquisitively, as I grabbed my stethoscope from the hook on the wall and took up my usual position of crawling around on my hands and knees on the consulting-room floor, face to face with my furred patient that was too large to feasibly lift onto the table.

The owner took a short break from tapping on her Blackberry handset. 'Yeah, she's pretty relaxed. You can do most things, she'll just stand there, like she's doing now.' She nodded her head towards Alice from her seat in the corner of the consulting room.

Alice's owner resumed arranging her schedule on her phone while I dutifully resumed my role on the floor. I followed the usual sequence, as all vets do, checking over each body system from nose, teeth, eyes, heart, chest, all the way to the tip of her tail. As I lay my two flattened palms on either side of Alice's abdomen, though, and started to palpate my way around, I noticed there was something present in the front part of her abdomen that shouldn't be there. Something huge. Bigger than both of my hands cupped together. Round, spherical, nodular and in the same region as the spleen, liver or possibly stomach. Imagine a pillowcase filled with raw bread dough and then a football being forced into

---

only we humans that stigmatise it. How confident can we be that if our own dogs were experiencing excruciating pain, they would not (understandably) resort to biting the hand that's trying to help them? I need my hands! Please don't ever be offended if a vet reasonably asks to place a muzzle on your dog for an examination.

the centre – you use your hands on the outside of the pillow-case to squidge and feel your way around the football – that is how it felt in Alice's abdomen.

Alice didn't flinch as I continued to gently work my fingertips and assess the size, shape and location of the mass. It didn't seem to be causing her any discomfort – and couldn't be seen from the outside as it was tucked partly up under her ribcage under her incredibly thick coat – but there was absolutely no doubt in my mind it was present. And it concerned me.

'Has she been off-colour at all lately? Any changes in her weeing or drinking, vomiting, diarrhoea? Has she been eating OK?' I rattled off a list of queries to see if I could inspire some engagement about Alice's recent general wellbeing.

'Errr, no. I don't think so. She's just normal – spends her time just sort of wandering around. We don't tend to walk her as much now – cos she's nine.' The owner placed her Blackberry onto her lap and brought her focus momentarily back into the room. 'She might be sleeping a bit more, but I just put that down to her age,' she continued. 'Why?'

'Well . . . I think . . . I can feel something in her abdomen.' I paused, and continued to feel and palpate Alice's tummy.

'Oh?'

'I'm pretty sure there is something . . . well, a mass . . . that seems to have grown on . . . *I'm guessing* . . . her liver or spleen,' I said while still feeling around Alice's abdomen. 'It could be an infection, or it could be a lymph node perhaps, but sadly, I think there is also quite a high chance' – this is the bit I always dread – 'that it could be cancerous.'

'Oh . . . right,' the owner replied quite plainly.

'I don't want to jump to any conclusions, though – I think

we should pop the scanner on her and then I should have a better idea of where it is and what it looks like. But I certainly don't think we should do her vaccinations today.'

The owner huffed with a frustrated impatience. I'd impressed her with my time-keeping punctuality, a strong start, but I'd ruined it all by throwing a huge curve ball into her precise schedule. I felt like my findings were a nuisance. A great nuisance which she really didn't need that day. That day of all days. 'I'm really sorry,' I said.

'Can you do the scan here?' she asked, pointing to the ground, 'here' referring to one of four branch practices to the main hospital.

'Yes, absolutely.'

'OK, fine,' she replied with efficient clarity. 'I'll have to call you next week as I'm away from now.' She looked at her watch as though she was working her day around a deadline, perhaps a train to catch.

'Err, well, yeah, we can do the scan for you here,' I replied confidently, 'although I'm thinking more like *today*.'

'Oh, bloody hell!' she muttered. The nuisance had now just mutated into a great big sledgehammer and smashed the diary in her Blackberry into a million tiny pieces.

I explained that if the mass was indeed on Alice's spleen, there was a risk it could spontaneously rupture. And if that happened, especially in the middle of the night or while Alice was on her own, it could quickly become life threatening and not be a pleasant way for her to go. She looked again at her watch. And that if the mass *was* on Alice's spleen, then we could potentially do a splenectomy (the surgical removal of the spleen). Whereas if it was on her liver, there would still be options available, but it may be something we'd need to

208

refer her to the main hospital for: a liver lobectomy, a biopsy or chemotherapy perhaps.

'Right,' she replied, taking a moment to consider her options. 'I just want you to be honest – it all sounds like what you're saying is this is *bad news*. Is it kinder for me to just put her down now?'

Even though I couldn't quite tell if this was a loaded question, knowing the owner had a train to catch, it was still a *fair* question. I had just found a probable tumour the size of a football in Alice's abdomen that could suddenly rupture at any point. If the bigger picture, with her busy lifestyle, was that any intervention was practically impossible, then euthanasia would be the only way I could guarantee Alice wouldn't suffer – and in that case, yes. But *I* felt that would be quite an extreme turn of events after arriving with an outwardly well Alice for her routine annual vaccination. The mass hadn't *yet* ruptured, and so perhaps there was a golden opportunity to intervene before it did so. If it weren't for the routine vaccination health check appointment, we would have remained none the wiser of the ticking time bomb that had silently grown within Alice, so perhaps this was the ticket we needed to get a step ahead of the game.

In the end the plan we agreed on was to leave Alice with me. I'd start with the ultrasound scan and Mrs Richardson would stay by her phone. Then, if it was a splenic mass, we had permission to take her to surgery. If it was a liver mass, with all things considered, she would prefer us to put Alice to sleep there and then and opt for a routine cremation. With that, the owner bent forwards from her chair, gave Alice a quick stroke over her head, said goodbye and then darted as fast as she could to catch her train. I felt Jackie Richardson was the kind of person who found comfort in having a plan. As long as there was a schedule to follow, she was OK. Still, only a quick pat on the head?

I led Alice to the kennels and settled her into a deep bed. After I'd finished up the morning consults, it was time to scan her abdomen. I clipped the fur from her belly, and with the help of a nurse to keep Alice still on the table in the darkened room, I placed the gelled probe onto her skin. A grainy grey and white pixellated moving image appeared on the screen. The smoother, more uniform texture of the spleen immediately differentiated itself from the more variable texture of the liver. Then a large, mottled irregular and unidentifiable structure erupted into view that looked suspiciously like cancer of her spleen, although it was impossible to tell on an ultrasound scan alone whether the cancer was benign or malignant.

By then it was around 2 p.m. I called Alice's owner. Her familiar voice answered: 'Hi, you've reached the voicemail of Jackie Richardson, please leave a message after the tone.'

With the realisation that my request to 'please stay by your phone' had fallen on deaf ears, I stifled a deep sigh of frustration and put my best professional phone voice on: 'Oh, hi there, it's James calling from the vet's. I've just scanned Alice and it is looking like the mass is on her spleen, so I'll follow through with the original plan and take her for surgery now, but feel free to call back if you want to discuss it further. Otherwise I'll give you another call when we are out of theatre. Thanks. Bye.'

I looked over at the nurse and shrugged my shoulders. I didn't really know what else to say. The nurse was eagerly awaiting permission to start prepping Alice for the anaesthetic. Despite having a signed consent form to go for surgery, I would still have preferred to have confirmation from her owner that she wanted me to perform this operation after our rushed consult first thing. But after fifteen minutes we'd still not heard; time was ticking and I was due to be consulting again at 3.30 p.m. I had the signed consent form so I made the decision: I'd take Alice to surgery.

A blood sample was taken from Alice's neck, which showed her vital parameters were within a normal range. We started Alice on a gentle rate of intravenous fluid therapy into her vein, which was shortly followed by the anaesthetic induction agent. Soon Alice was lying on her back in the operating theatre. The rhythmic beeping sound of the multi-parameter machine told the anaesthetic nurse that everything was stable. Then, dressed in a surgeon's hat, gloves and gown, I hovered my scalpel blade over the naked, shaved skin of Alice's belly. The nurse gave a nod to begin, and I ran the blade along the pink skin from the point just beneath the end of her ribcage to the mid-point of her abdomen. After entering through the abdominal muscle layer, the huge mass was immediately apparent. Sitting just beneath the surface, it was at least the size of a football. A football that was, indeed, attached to the spleen, *thankfully*. Silent and deadly, an ever-expanding, mottled, deep maroon and black coloured mass that looked moments away from popping, like an overstretched water balloon.

I've always felt like the spleen is a somewhat redundant addition to a dog's anatomy, an afterthought. A name on the second round of invites to a wedding. Of course, in reality it isn't – and does have a vitally important function as a blood filtration service to regulate the body's immune defences

211

– but it always baffles me how animals can (and do) seem to cope so very well without it. It makes you ponder what the merit is for the spleen to be there in the first place, for all the trouble it causes. The whole organ can be removed, shelled from the body like a spare part without requiring any long-term medication afterwards, and in cases like Alice's, dogs are often all the better for it. The question, though, is for how long?

There are a few reasons why a spleen could swell: it could be due to a malignant tumour called a haemangiosarcoma; a benign tumour of the vessels called a haemangioma; a huge blood clot within the spleen called a haematoma, or a plethora of infectious agents that could cause an abscess. As there is a risk of rupture, taking any sort of biopsy prior to surgery can be very tricky, as there is a distinct risk we may 'pop' the balloon or 'seed' the cancerous cells around the body as the needle is withdrawn. Therefore, as long as there is no evidence of concurrent cancer spread on the ultrasound scan, it is often deemed appropriate to go ahead and remove the spleen first and then attempt to diagnose the mass retrospectively on histology. It's the one time we often have no choice but to make a diagnosis 'in hindsight' – normally, especially with cancer surgery, we like to know exactly what we are dealing with before we put an animal through a procedure. The age-old 'is it fair?' debate. But in the case of a spleen, we tend to do the surgery first and make the diagnosis second because in all cases it will almost certainly save the dog's life, at least in the short run.

'Woah, it's massive,' I said to the nurse as I ran my hands around the surface of the nodular growth. 'We're going to need more artery forceps . . . and extra swabs.' The nurse nodded and went to retrieve some more sterile packs of instruments. *Count. Your. Swabs*, the inner voice in my head repeated over and over as the nurse opened countless packs of white cotton swabs and metal surgical instruments. Counting the surgical instrumentation and swabs in *and out* of a patient's abdomen is a key lesson in veterinary surgery. There is no greater panic than trying to work out if there is a missing swab or an escaped forcep in the cavernous abdomen of a large dog on the very last stitch at the very end of a very long and complicated surgery.

I started the methodical process of steadily working my way around the vessels and attachments of the spleen. Clamp, ligate, clamp, cut, repeat. Clamp, ligate, clamp, cut, repeat.

It helps if there is another vet or nurse scrubbed in to help manoeuvre the spleen, but such a luxury was not on offer. I was on my tod. Eventually, I double ligated the last, large vessel and with one final slice of my blade, the cancerous football was cut free from Alice's body. I lifted the spleen and accompanying mass out of the cavernous abdomen and dropped it into a stainless-steel bowl at the end of the operating table. The bowl chimed as the metal clamps tinkled against it, like a musical bell to mark the removal of Alice's tumour. It was huge. I looked back down at Alice, who suddenly seemed to have shrunk by a third of her original size and checked over the rest of her inners looking for any signs of tumour spread.

'Jeeeez!' the receptionist suddenly appeared at the theatre window and spotted the mass from outside the theatre. She mouthed through the glass pane, 'James, just to let you know Mrs Richardson just phoned back . . .'

'An hour later!' I replied, concerned about what may come next, as I continued to suture the final muscle layer and finish closing up. 'Go on?'

'She said to go ahead with the surgery . . . which I can see . . . is good news!' The receptionist smiled and tilted her head towards the solid organ sitting in the stainless-steel bowl, like a giant haggis in a butcher's window. We glanced a look of relief to each other.

Alice recovered well from her surgery. She stayed overnight and her owner returned the following day, this time with a slightly less rushed approach to life. I talked her through the aftercare, the need for rest, the pain relief I was sending Alice home on and the necessity to prevent her from licking the wound by equipping her with the dreaded 'cone of shame'. I commented on how well Alice had done, and how she had been the model patient for our nursing team to care for. I reassured her that I'd call with the final prognosis once I had the histology results back from the veterinary pathologists and that the final invoice was within estimate, as agreed. Everything was just as it should be.

This is often the moment there is some owner jubilation, relief that their beloved companion is safe, that they had survived a huge operation and get to go home. But for Alice, the reunion triggered no celebration, no hug or stroke of the head, no real display of *any* emotion. Alice's owner took the lead from my hand, said a moderate thank you, asked how much the final bill was, paid without quibble and left. It all felt very 'transactional'.

A week later, I reported the results. It was in fact a haemangioma, the more favourable and arguably least probable of the various possibilities. Good news – we had undoubtedly

214

bought Alice many extra months if not years compared to a 'do nothing' approach. All on the back of a routine vaccination health check appointment. Though again our conversation was brief, flat and succinct. The owner thanked me and swiftly hung up. And that was that.

I can remember feeling quite despondent that Alice's owner had not felt more elated by this outcome. Normally, reporting that a patient was cancer-free was a massive highlight, a celebration between myself and my client, that together we had 'beaten cancer' for their pet. I was maybe only five years into my career and had felt the prompt diagnosis and surgical treatment, all within the same day, was quite an epic achievement. It *was* an achievement and, in hindsight, I *was* right to feel quietly proud of the work the team had performed. I suppose, though, to some, at the end of the day I was also just *doing my job*. I didn't perform the surgery on Alice for the praise of her owner, I did it for Alice. And if the praise hadn't come externally, then I had to learn to be comfortable with that. The cards, the wine, the chocolates are all hugely motivating, extremely kind gestures of thanks – and do mean such a great deal to the team when they arrive – but I could not let that define my enjoyment of working as a vet.

A few weeks later a card did arrive in the post, addressed to myself and the team. There was a cartoon figure of a dog on the front holding a flag with the words 'Thank you' written across it. In it, Alice's owner wrote how grateful she was for the team's care, how much it had meant to her that we had discovered the mass and how pleased she was that we found it before it had ruptured. She shared that she too had been diagnosed a few years previously and had overcome her own personal battle with cancer, and how the two of them were now 'survivors together'. As I read the card, everything suddenly made sense.

I realised then that I can never know everything that is going on with a client, nor have I any right to expect that I should. Some people will choose to share, others will not, but whatever the case, how those people react in a situation doesn't necessarily give the whole picture. Whether that's a person saying thank you, or a person hurling abuse, there is nearly always an explanation and often more to a situation than may meet the eye. Veterinary medicine is extremely grounding in that respect.

At veterinary school we had been given some practical sessions to help hone our 'communication skills', but these were primarily aimed at how to *deliver* sad news. All very useful stuff, as a starting point. But what next? I felt confident in how to find a way to deliver a diagnosis: to remain factual, scientific and honest. The real challenge for me has always been in the small pause while the headline news sinks in and I await their reaction. And every pet owner responds differently. It's one thing to deliver the news but what is *their* response going to be back to me? And how do I take the conversation on from there? You can try to sugarcoat it, wrap it up in soft language, focus on the positives, but at the end of the day, it's just never going to be pleasant for a pet owner to hear the news they may have been dreading the most. Diagnosing pets with cancer is, I think, perhaps the most emotive subject of all.

We probably all know of someone, maybe even someone close, who has sadly lost their battle with cancer. There is a generalised anxiety associated with cancer; even just the word can trigger a fear within all of us. And cancer in our pets brings with it a whole unique set of concerns for owners. On the one hand, it is a relief that pets don't have the emotional capability to understand their own diagnosis, and therefore don't share the same concept of their own projected time or prognosis. On the other hand, it throws up many ethical considerations around what to treat, how to treat and even *whether* to treat the cancer.

I was halfway through one consultation when just at the very mention of the word 'cancer', as a vague possibility in a long list of potential differentials regarding a dog's painful lameness, the owner raised both his hands and kindly insisted that I stopped talking. He fought through choked emotion to form his words and explained that only three days previously, he had lost his wife to an aggressive form of breast cancer, within a matter of weeks of diagnosis, which had occurred only a month before they were both due to retire. 'It's the part of life you're supposed to enjoy after working so bloody hard,' he said with his head in his hands, 'and now it's been taken from us both.'

I'll never forget it. I could feel the intense sorrow, trapped in the four walls of my small consultation room. His wife, who was the one who would usually have accompanied their dogs on a trip to the vet's and who I'd seen many times over the previous years, was completely delightful. I didn't have a clue what to say. These moments are astonishingly intimate; they are close, palpable and they stay with you. I felt and shared his sorrow. And still, somehow, I had to navigate my way around discussing what the options were to investigate his eight-year-old Bernese mountain dog that had presented with a painful, swollen joint, within a fifteen-minute consult-ation, fully aware I also had a full waiting room outside. I can't recall ever being taught how to communicate your way through any of *that*. I suppose it was just expected that a vet will learn to cope.

I have always worked in general practice. I am a GP vet. I have seen every walk of life step through my consulting-room door, witnessed every demographic: every age group; people with differing sexualities; differing genders; differing races and religions; differing mental health challenges and differing financial circumstances. Many, many different rep-resentations of life. And the commonality that links all these different people together is that the vast majority simply want advice on how to do 'what's best' for their pets.

Choosing what is best, though, is not always clear-cut. It is too binary. If there is a best option, that suggests there is a worst option. The same with right or wrong. If one option presented is deemed to be the 'brave' one, does that make the alternative option cowardly?

Language is a powerfully persuasive tool. Subtle words or phrases can really sway a person's decision-making process and that brings with it huge responsibility when it comes to treating a person's pet. Bravery can display itself in many forms in my consulting room. It is incredibly brave to put a pet through any surgery. But, in my eyes, the caveat of *any* surgery is that it has to be an improvement to the overall quality and longevity of an animal's life for that individual. To put an animal through major surgery just because we can, or without known proof or expectation that it will improve the outcome afterwards, I'd ask, is that being 'brave' or is that actually quite selfish – to put an individual animal

218

through something so major without much proven benefit to them? As vets, we find ourselves treading that fine line daily, attempting to define what is 'best' for a pet and often making that decision comes down to trust. Trust between the vet and the pet owner to weigh up the pros and cons and make that decision together.

Some owners are adamant they won't even entertain the idea of putting their pet through chemotherapy. They'll say they 'don't agree with it' before I have even had a chance to explain. Others want to do everything, absolutely everything, and disregard my concerns that it may not *necessarily* be in the best interests of their pet.

I have seen incredible results with chemotherapy and with cancer surgery. I have seen dogs literally trot into the surgery desperately happy to see everyone and enjoy the handful of treats while we get dressed up looking like forensic scientists and administer the chemotherapy injection. I've known placid cats fall asleep during treatment. The mast cell tumour that sat inoperably close to a dog's jugular vein shrank and then disappeared for almost three years of joyful remission on a daily chemotherapy tablet. Expensive, yes, but without doubt a huge success as an example of treating cancer with chemotherapy in our pets. A lymph node the size of a tangerine disappeared for thirteen months, buying the happiest cat (who loved coming in for his cuddles and occasional chemo appointment) many extra, happy months. I've removed countless skin lumps that have been sent in formalin to the pathologist with confirmed margins of excision and never knowingly regrown. And I can say for certain that many lives have been lovingly extended through referral to our specialist veterinary oncologists. Where the land lies when it comes to treating cancer in our pets is hugely variable. It depends on a whole myriad of factors. Committing to a chemotherapy schedule, though, is a huge decision.

I was once asked the question whether I thought veterinary medicine had gone 'too far'. And whether some of the media portrayal of veterinary medicine meant there was pressure on pet owners to put their pets through more than they're comfortable with. I turned the question back on the pet owner, interested to hear his opinion. He said he thought we had lost all common sense, that animals are no longer treated as animals and instead we see them the same way we do humans, and as a result vets' bills have become unaffordably expensive, as has insurance, as we take their treatment too far. He would do it for his child, but not for his dog. It was certainly a thought-provoking question.

My answer then, and still now, is that what works for one person and their pet won't necessarily be the same for another. And I think the wonderful thing about veterinary medicine is that we do have such a huge freedom of individual choice. To choose the path that suits best.

As GP vets, we can tailor our approach to your pet's care in many different ways – from offering basic medication and ensuring an animal is not in pain, to referring a pet to a specialist centre for the most advanced surgical procedures to remove brain tumours, 'cure' cancers, replace arthritic hip joints or even fit a bionic limb. But of course, at other times, it may be that the time has come to offer a gentle, peaceful end. The spectrum of options available for our pets these days is vast. For me, being a GP vet is about helping a pet owner choose the most suitable option at the time for them and their pet, but that doesn't mean taking your pet's treatment to a level you are not comfortable with. Just because we can do something doesn't mean we should, or that we have to. How far someone chooses to take treatment is ultimately up to the pet owner under their own individual circumstances. My only one strong opinion is that there is never, ever any justification to leave an animal suffering in pain.

And in fact, many times I hear 'seasoned' pet owners confess that they regret some of the choices they made with their first pet. They recognise they were never coerced into making decisions against their will, but in hindsight, having been through an interventional process with their pets, they felt they *had* taken things too far. Sometimes I'm even faced with an owner who has solemnly vowed to themselves that they simply wouldn't be putting their next pet through the same level of treatment. And while I can empathise with that, I do also think every animal, every treatment plan and every outcome will be individual to *that* animal and should be approached as such. Caring for a pet is a huge responsibility and making informed choices can feel overwhelming. But with so many options available, instead of seeing that as a negative, I think we should see it as an opportunity for each of us to choose our own path for our own pets. And no matter how apprehensive or confused things may feel in the moment, I can guarantee that in every situation, there should nearly always be more than one treatment option for you to consider.

CHAPTER 12

Nala

(This chapter contains a description of severe animal cruelty and abuse that may be distressing.)

It was just one of those days. The kind of day that is hard to decipher. There is no rhyme or reason to them, but every GP vet will know exactly what I am talking about.

It started with a lovely cockerpoo, Monty, with an equally lovely but completely chaotic owner who somehow managed to live her life ten minutes late for everything. A notorious repeat offender, I had never known her arrive on time, ever – but she had always been so charming with it that no one really knew how to address it with her. And so, instead, we'd usually reserve a slot for her at the end of a consulting block, rather than the beginning. A sort of 'damage limitation without offending her' tactic. But our new receptionist wasn't privy to this secret code on 'how to manage Monty and his chaotic mum' and had instead booked her the 9 a.m. consultation.

The mistake had gone unnoticed, too late was the cry. Already 9.04 and there was no sign of either of them. She usually turned up wearing a long floaty skirt, flip-flops and wet combed-through hair that carried the strong scent of coconut conditioner and chlorine from her morning swim. A huge, brightly coloured, woven bag would be flung over her right shoulder that carried everything she might need to get through her manic schedule and Monty would be trotting along quite patiently beside her. Despite having a million things on her mind, for someone whose life was pure chaos she always managed to look as though she'd just stepped off the beach.

Monty really was very sweet. As a vet, I do not have favourite patients – all dogs and cats are truly amazing. But there are some that just somehow manage to get a little closer. I had seen Monty for his first vaccinations as a puppy when I started at the practice, and we had kind of 'grown up' together. I had answered the long list of questions the family had scribbled on a piece of A4 paper as worried, first-time dog owners. And I had seen him every year since for his boosters. Given tips on how to soothe his itching skin in the summer months and had been on hand to make him vomit when – for some unknown reason – he decided to gobble down one of the children's sports socks. I even held his ears back while the regurgitated stomach contents splattered over me, my nurse and the consulting-room walls when he shook his head mid-wretch. I returned the sock in a plastic bag. And, in return, out of their eternal gratitude, I received a huge tray of Green and Black's posh chocolate with a card that read: 'Dear James, hope these look more appetising than the sock did! Love Monty x'

I really liked them and had got to know Monty well. But it was now 9.08 and my next client – not the kind of man who liked to be kept waiting – was due for a 9.15 appointment with Jax, his Jack Russell terrier that had started the morning passing bright red, bloody diarrhoea. As the clock ticked to 9.10, I took a quick look at the 'financials' tab at the top right-hand corner of my computer screen. On Monty alone, they had already spent £7,956 over the past eighteen months, a quarter of my annual salary. Monty suffered with terrible allergies; his was a complicated case that required extensive management and the appointment on that day had been booked in under the heading 'Skin flare-up, eyes not right'. Eventually, at 9.11, Monty came happily trotting across the car park, unaware of the huge, bright bag swaying precariously over his head. 'I'm so sorry I'm late,' I overheard from reception.

I picked up the handset on the phone and dialled through to reception. The new voice answered, 'Hello, veterinary practice, how can I help you?'

'No, no, it's James in room one,' I replied. 'I'm just about to call Monty in but can you explain to Jax's owner when he arrives that I'm running ten minutes late and will be with him as soon as possible?' I tried to stay upbeat, but felt for her own sake I should also give her a heads-up, to pre-empt his probable reaction. 'He can be a little bit sharp, just to warn you!'

Only ten minutes late would be a miracle. I knew Monty would probably need at least twenty minutes and there was no other vet in the building for another hour. My fate was sealed. I'd be running twenty minutes behind for every appointment thereafter, playing catch-up as I worked my way through the long list of fully booked fifteen-minute appointments. We were in a busy phase – quite why a vet's practice would go through busy or quiet phases, I've never really understood. Of course, there are the occasional outbreaks of kennel cough, or tummy upsets that go around, and we might see a small spike in appointments for a few days. But this wasn't that. The phone had been ringing off the hook for the past few weeks – vaccination appointments, new puppy appointments, lame pets, vomiting pets, pets with diarrhoea, pets with ear infections, pets that weren't quite right, pets that were travelling abroad. And even more would phone in.

The new voice appeared on the end of the internal telephone again. 'Hi, it's Jane again. I've had to squeeze you an extra one in, James – Dillon, the cat you saw last night, now hasn't peed at all in his tray but keeps straining. They said you told them to call if that happened.' A male cat that can't pass urine is an emergency. When male cats get 'blocked' the urine collects in the bladder which causes back pressure up to the kidneys, electrolyte changes, severe kidney damage and even death. 'There aren't any appointments left so I've just booked him in at the end. Is that OK?'

I politely explained that would be too late and instead to phone them back and tell them to come straight down. As well as itchy Monty turning up late, I'd also admitted Jax the Jack Russell passing blood from his back end (and tempered his very disgruntled owner) and now had to find a way to squeeze in a blocked Dillon, who would very likely require blood tests and a sedation to pass a urinary catheter to relieve his bladder. This was on top of the three procedures written up on the board – a bitch spay, a rabbit dental and a 'sedate to check ears'. I put the phone down and watched any hope of a lunch break, or any break, disappear down the sink as I washed my hands and prepared to call my next patient in.

Of course, as a vet I don't ever begrudge the pets themselves, or their caring owners who are doing the dutiful thing and phoning for help and guidance. This is what we love doing, it is why we became vets. But when the days overflow, it can feel that there is no time to rejoice in success or grieve at the sad times, because the roller coaster never stops. You are constantly making decisions and calling the shots and the intensity continues day after day. Even a brave face can only last so long.

This was one of those such days. The energy, at first, can be quite addictive, quite buzzy. But after a while, that energy can turn to anxiety. The constant fear of trying to keep up, keep going, trying to stay focused, delegate to the nursing team (who have been understaffed for months) and all the while not let anyone down. I had to treat Dillon the emergency around the fully booked consults, called in favours from friends for advice, pinged an email with X-rays attached for a second opinion on a lame dog, pinged another email to a referral centre to chase the report for another dog whose liver they'd partially removed and who was due to come for a check-up in less than an hour. Some call it 'ducking' – serene up top with legs flapping furiously underneath. I was paddling as hard as I could, but it had started to feel like my duck was slowly sinking.

This was also the kind of day where I found myself apologising all day long. Saying I'm sorry to the three clients who had been kept waiting in reception due to an unforeseen emergency. Saying I'm sorry to the nursing team who give 'that look' when I showed up with Dillon while they were still triaging Jax. Saying I'm sorry to the animals themselves who are in a state of shock, nausea, trauma or pain and unable to comprehend or understand why or what was going on. Saying I'm sorry to my vet colleague who eventually turned up for their half day of work to find we had the work of three full-time vets to somehow battle through. And saying I'm sorry to the heartbroken couple whose elderly beagle I had to put to sleep at the end of the day.

Almost everyone is understanding. But despite everyone doing their best, these busy days can also lead to tensions and disappointments. These are the days that can make it feel like you are no longer thriving, you're not even coping. You're just firefighting. And all the while trying to make sure you don't make a monumental cock-up.

I followed consults with surgery and then finally, by mid-afternoon, I'd caught up enough to find ten minutes to wolf down a sarnie. But as I calmed the grumbling pit of my stomach with a bite of an anaemic-looking sandwich from the nearby petrol station, the receptionist appeared once again at the staffroom door. 'Don't hate me, James,' she said in a kind of cartoon and apologetically high-pitched voice, 'but we've had another walk-in.'

I replaced my half-eaten sandwich in the paper packaging and said farewell to my lunch break.

'I did ask them to take a seat, but he said he wanted to see a vet now. He said it's an emergency. I didn't recognise them, though; I don't *think* we've ever seen them before.'

I followed her into the reception waiting area and picked the last few strands of tuna mayonnaise from my teeth with my tongue. We were greeted by two men standing squarely in the middle of the reception area, with a mass of fur held in the arms of one. I always find there's something quite telling about a person who chooses to *not* take a seat when they have been invited to do so. Maybe they're in shock, upset or seriously worried about their pet. An emergency, perhaps. Or they're being polite, they've just popped in and don't want to overstay their welcome if they just want a 'quick answer' to a simple question. Or, sometimes, they just don't want to be *told* what to do – they're primed with adrenaline, perhaps ready to make a complaint. Either way, a person that chooses to remain standing in a room full of empty chairs usually tells me *something* is about to kick off.

I introduced myself and asked them to come through to the consulting room. The two men were in their late twenties. The slightly younger-looking one lowered the mound of fur from his arms and placed it onto the consulting-room table. It took a moment for me to realise it was in fact a dog as the thick, matted fur had clumped into long woven locks of dirt and neglect that hung like strands of thick rope covering the entire body surface of the animal – her legs, back end and face. The smell was intense. A farm smell of dried manure. Then I spotted her front left leg was tied with multiple ribbons of a ripped-up tea towel. It had been wrapped and tightened around the circumference of the leg, strapped onto a plank of one-inch squared MDF wood. 'It's just happened,' he said, 'dunno how.'

I put on a pair of latex gloves and started to unravel the makeshift splint. As I removed each subsequent layer of tea towel, soiled wood shavings fell from the inner layers of the dressing. Eventually, the wet plank of old wood collapsed, like a felled tree, onto the consult table and made a loud 'clang' as I loosened the last strap holding it in place. The dog released a small yelp and tried to walk to the edge of the table. She held her leg off the ground. A dog in pain can react a million different ways, including having to resort to aggression, but up to that point she had been remarkably passive and accepting.

I paused and stroked the top of her head. 'I'm sorry,' I apologised to her.

Her tail wagged ferociously, and her tongue began to lick the air. She couldn't see out from the matted fur hanging from the brow of her eyes, but once she had managed to locate my hand, she licked it, over and over, while her tail spun like a helicopter in overdrive. At that point, I realised, through the innocence of her reaction, that she was still young. Perhaps even still a puppy. 'How old is she?' I asked.

'Dunno, she's my aunt's dog,' he replied.

'Ahh, OK,' I replied. *The smell of bullshit had now also filled the air.* I continued to undress the leg. And eventually reached the final layer of towelling. The cotton fabric had soaked into a wound that appeared to stretch at least four inches along the length of her leg. The fabric, though, had been there some time, as the portion in contact with the open wound had dried to a solid crust. I attempted to free one edge, but she yelped again, only this time louder. And then resorted again to her submissive air licking and tail wagging.

'You say this has just happened?'

'Yeah, mate, just now. She was playing with another dog.'

No chance, I thought to myself. 'We'll need to contact your aunt,' I replied, pulling the latex gloves from my hands. 'I'm going to need to sedate her for me to remove the dressing and work out what's going on.'

The men looked at each other.

'Can we give her a call?' I asked, while looking at the wound.

'She's not available,' the larger of the two men replied, 'she told us to just do whatever.'

'OK, but if this is her dog, I *am* going to need her permission before I can do anything.'

'She's gone on holiday.'

'Does she have a phone number?'

'No.'

'Right,' I replied, trying to mentally flick through the veterinary rule book in my mind on how the hell I'm meant to navigate around gaining consent. 'Well, I'll still need to register you as a client first and then, I guess, if you're happy to sign on her behalf?'

'Yeah, yeah, she's my dog anyway.'

What?

'She's my dog so I can sign it, yeah. She just lives with my aunt.'

I printed off a consent form and the young man signed it. He declined to offer a phone number. And wrote 'Nala' as the dog's name, then scribbled what turned out to be a false address.

I talked them through my proposed plan, to sedate Nala, assess and clean the wound and then potentially either suture her leg or come up with a way to manage the wound. The man agreed to the estimate and said he would return at 5 p.m. to collect her. We parted and I took the juvenile mound of fur round the back to the practice prep area. The smell of cow faeces, with the clumps of her own faeces mingled with the tarry bitumen smell of TCP antiseptic wafted from the stuck-down scrap of tea towel soaked into her leg wound. Yet, despite all of whatever it was that she had been through at the hands of humans, Nala was a completely delightful young dog. I placed her on the prep table and the team of nurses came over to meet her.

'I think she's still a puppy,' I said, above the sound of many hearts breaking as the nursing team all 'ooh'd' and 'ahh'd' over the poor state of this young pup. I scanned her for a microchip. Knowing if there had been a chip present, and it was registered, things could get very complicated. Perhaps Nala had been stolen? Was there a family somewhere in desperate hope of being reunited? But there was no microchip.

The nursing team distracted Nala by allowing her to lick their hands and climb up them to reach their faces. They wrapped their arms around her, despite her farmyard odour, while I placed a cannula into her leg vein. She immediately melted all our hearts. And then I administered a sedative medication to allow me to tend to her wounded leg. As she drifted into a quiet slumber, and a face mask delivered a gentle flow of oxygenated air for her to breathe deeply, I continued to remove the layer of crusted tea towel. Knowing the pain was no longer registering in Nala's nervous system, thanks to her sedation, I dowsed the fabric with diluted iodine solution before peeling back the corner of the dressing to break through the sealed crust. As I pulled the cotton fabric away from her exposed wound, a green snotty discharge that had accumulated beneath poured out but the blood that oozed was a deep maroon colour, not the bright red blood of a fresh wound, confirming my suspicion that the injury had not 'just happened'.

As I continued to peel, though, the full horrifying extent

of the open wound came to light. Through the dark, stagnant pool of stale blood, and the green pus that had collected around the margins of the wound, two shards of white bone protruded through her open skin. Her leg was fractured, snapped in two like a stick. The pain must have been excruciating. 'Jeez,' I said to the nurse assisting me, who was also looking on with absolute horror. 'How long have they left it like that?'

The nurse, Tom, carried Nala through to the X-ray room. The radiograph soon appeared on the screen and showed us the full extent of her injury. A full thickness fracture across the radius and ulna, the two bones of her foreleg, only an inch or so away from her carpus (or wrist joint). Snapped, clean in two. The diagonal fracture line had displaced the bones left and right of each other.

'What shall we do?' Tom asked.

'Well,' I replied, 'she's still a puppy, so probably still got some growing to do and now she has an infected open fracture. I've got no phone numbers. I don't even know who the bloody owner is. And I've got no idea if those two men are even going to come back.'

I pulled both my hands up through my hair and stood, staring at the X-ray image of the young puppy in front of me. The bill had already reached the top end of the estimate I had given them, but with the radiograph in front of me, this was just the tip of the iceberg. 'OK, well, let's take a swab from the wound, and start her on some antibiotics tonight – we can't do anything until that infection is under control,' I said, still staring at the radiograph. Tom cleaned the wound and then packed a clear wound gel into the exposed tissue, before placing a sturdy dressing over her leg.

Five o'clock soon came but the two men who had dropped Nala off were nowhere to be seen. Nala had recovered from her sedation and quickly guzzled down a full bowl of food in a matter of seconds, so we settled her in with a deep bed and she stayed overnight – drifting in and out of her hazy, opiate-infused, dream-filled sleep, unsure whether the two men would ever return.

The following day the men did show up. I showed them the radiographs and explained the situation: that I had discovered a fracture (which I suspect they already knew as it explained why they had attempted to strap a piece of wood to her leg), and that the wound was already deeply infected. She would certainly need referral to orthopaedic surgery if we had any chance of saving the leg.* I explained that referral would likely cost upwards of three grand, and as they didn't have pet insurance, the referral practice would probably require payment in full. Amputation was another option – cheaper, but very final. It would perhaps seem a shame to lose the leg of a young dog when the fracture itself was potentially operable, but we had already run over the estimate, due to the unforeseen overnight stay, and I had to be realistic that cost does often play a deciding factor in these situations. As an employed vet, it's not unusual to be on the sharp end of some snide remarks around the cost of veterinary medicine, as though I somehow have the power to change the figure (I can't) or see a share of the profits (I don't).†

---

* Ideally, with this sort of fracture, we would perform surgery within twenty-four to forty-eight hours of the accident happening. I suspected that window had long gone and was keen for a specialist surgeon to help decide the best route of action.

† The cost of veterinary medicine to an owner is set by the business

But these two men just nodded. 'Nah, I can't see her on only three legs, Doc, doesn't seem fair,' he said. I wanted to remind him that strapping a piece of wood to a dog's fractured leg and leaving them for days in pain *isn't fair*, but in the hope of reaching a solution for Nala, I managed to bite my tongue. Fortunately, I had painted a bleak enough picture that they seemed to comprehend that Nala couldn't be left simply as she was and they agreed that referral would be the best option. 'Just take her for the surgery,' he said.

This was by far the best solution for Nala and, as long

---

owner – whether a private equity firm, joint venture, corporate practice or an independent – not the employed vet in the consult room. As with the majority of business models, there are a proportionally small number people at the top of the tree, making extortionate amounts of money out of the veterinary industry. To try to suggest otherwise would be an insult to both vets on the ground and the pet-owning public that fork out thousands for their pets' care. But to provide a fully equipped private healthcare service (which is, essentially, what veterinary medicine is) requires huge investment and running costs. A CT scanner, for example, costs tens of thousands of pounds to the practice. That money has to come in from somewhere. There is no government funding, there is no NHS for pets. But for how expensive veterinary care may seem, it is important to consider that it is not *all profit*. In fact, the profit margins in veterinary medicine are notoriously pretty tight. The huge majority goes on all the fixed costs – such as rent, investment in equipment, utility bills, insurances, consumables such as drugs and of course wages to pay the staff. And, as a result, the average employed GP vet or vet nurse you meet in the consulting room will likely be on far lower salaries than the public often perceive. And while veterinary turnover is often monitored by business owners or external management consultancy firms, it is very unusual for vets to be rewarded individually for their turnover or to receive a financial 'bonus' of any kind as incentive for their individual clinical work or decision-making.

as they followed the post-operative care, then the overall prognosis was good. Despite the infection, I was cautiously optimistic that Nala's leg could still be saved. A plan in place, I left the two men and began phoning around the various referral practices to see if I could find a price. A few hours later, we were meeting back in reception again.

'All right, mate,' they agreed. 'Yeah, just do whatever you need to do.'

'Great,' I said, leaving them to settle up the outstanding invoice as I went to confirm the referral. But then, once again, things shifted. The receptionist came to find me. 'James, they've asked if they can speak with you again.'

What? Why? I walked through to reception.

'Oi, Doc.' The younger man caught me as I walked in. 'Yeah, I spoke wiv my aunt and she said to just put her down.'

WHAT?

'She said it's not worth spending that sort of money so to just put her down instead.'

Are you kidding me?

'What about amputation? If you can't go for referral?' I asked.

He shrugged his shoulders.

I ran through the options again. They even refused the idea of charity assistance, which would have required multiple ID checks and paperwork. I asked what they might be able to afford, even just as a contribution towards amputation – or whether a payment plan could work. But again they declined and said they 'didn't want to have to look at a three-legged dog'. They then told the receptionist they couldn't (or wouldn't) pay the outstanding amount. It became clear that

FOR THE LOVE OF ANIMALS

they never had any intention of handing over any money from the get-go. Clearly the two lads had planned to walk in, get their dog fixed, promise to pay later, and instead disappear. But their plan hadn't worked and now they just wanted the problem gone.

But in my mind euthanasia was simply not an option. There was no way I was going to put Nala to sleep for something entirely fixable. But if I were to decline their request, I also couldn't legally stop them from taking Nala home, insisting they would find another vet that *would* perform the euthanasia or worse – take matters into their own hands. I didn't want to hand Nala back to them. We had reached a stalemate. It left only one other option to consider: relinquish their ownership. The two men could sign Nala over and hand all decision-making and financial burden to the practice. The trade-off was that they would not be able to request Nala back. We would absorb the cost of all work (or rather, my boss and the practice would), Nala would become our responsibility and eventually we would find her a suitable new home. It is a lot of work for a practice to take on, and a huge financial burden. In these morally conflicting situations, though, it is sometimes the only lifeline we have left to offer an animal in need.

I feel it is worth saying a couple of things here. Firstly, vets are not in the game of taking animals off owners who can't afford vets' bills. There are always options – from gold-standard care down to the most basic intervention. And there are options around how to cover costs. As a vet, I see it as my role to explore these options with an individual owner and find a solution. There are times, though, where we are on different pages, as was the case with Nala. Euthanasia is as much at my discretion to offer as it is for an owner to simply request. Euthanasia was their definite and final choice, but it was not mine. And in these rare cases, the owner has already decided to part ways with their pet; they have already said goodbye. It didn't make much difference to these two men what happened to Nala, they just wanted to wash their hands of her – sounds cold, and perhaps scathing of me to say it, but it is true. In my mind, though, signing Nala over was win-win. I can even temper my anger in these situations as, deep down, through signing her over they did at least give her a chance of a future.

On the other hand, what does *really* anger me as a vet is that there's absolutely nothing to stop these men from using the money saved on the vet's fees for Nala to simply go out and buy another puppy on a whim.

Nonetheless, with the situation in front of me, I pitched the idea of signing Nala over to us and, without any hesitation, he signed the paperwork. He thanked me, even shook my hand and we never saw either of them again. I walked back through to the prep area. These highly emotive scenarios are often felt through the entire team and the nurses had dreaded me coming back with the news that the men were going to either take Nala home or, even worse, insist on putting her to sleep. When I shared the news, there was a deep sigh of relief. Everyone had fallen for Nala, and now there was a chance we could make her better. But it did leave me with one very harsh realisation – I had just taken on the sole responsibility for an untrained puppy, who I guessed was only about ten months old, with a broken leg and an unknown future.

A few hours later I returned again to find Nala standing

on the prep table surrounded by the nursing team and a selection of scissors, combs, brushes and other pet grooming paraphernalia. The monotone sound of the handheld electric clippers whizzed and buzzed as they ploughed through her matted coat. And with each few inches, another clump of rope-like matted fur fell to the ground and carpeted the lino surgery floor. Her fringe of matted hair had been trimmed away and for the first time, her big chocolate eyes glistened. As her tail started to wag ferociously, her bottom waggled from side to side in her trademark move as our eyes met for the very first time.

'Hello, gorgeous!' I said as I stepped towards the table. She took two or three steps towards me and then started licking as I reached out to cup her chin in my hand and stroke over her new fresh-faced head of hair.

'Oi, stop distracting her!' Kym the nurse giggled as she tried to regain control of the exuberant puppy bouncing on the table in front of her. 'She's not finished her makeover yet!'

It took four applications of some strawberry-scented doggy suds to rid her of the smell of farm manure, but as the water trickled from her coat like a muddy brown river of sewage, gradually a brand-new Nala emerged. Underneath her thick coat of neglect we discovered a poodle-crossed-spanielly-looking puppy with a caramel-coloured undercoat and a large white blaze across her chest. She looked a good few kilograms lighter too, which made the hefty lime-green bandage on her front left leg seem even more cumbersome.

'She looks so good!' I said, with a huge smile to Kym. The transformation was extraordinary. 'I still haven't a clue what we're going to do with that leg, though,' I added, as the team all marvelled at Nala's new look.

Referral was pretty much out of the question, as it would have meant the practice picking up the bill of thousands of pounds. I could, of course, beg and plead for a discount, but it felt a little perverse to take on Nala as our responsibility and then pass the financial debt on to another vet's practice. Amputation is simple enough surgery – you basically just keep cutting – but I felt frustrated by my own clinical limitations that I couldn't do more than just hack her leg off. The fracture was fixable, but no one in the practice (myself included) had any real experience in performing orthopaedic surgery. We tended to refer all our orthopaedic cases to a nearby specialist. Physics was never my strong suit at school – I could never get my head around loading, bending or pulling forces – so orthopaedics, which is basically all about angles and forces and weight bearing, never really held much interest. It also involves drills. And while I hate to play to any stereotypes, I'm not *the best* when it comes to DIY. Orthopaedics is all nuts and bolts, drills and screws, metal rods and plates. If you were the kind of child who loved the challenge of a complicated Meccano kit, orthopaedics would be for you. Sadly, I was not that child!

'You should do it!' Kym replied.

'Eh?'

'You should do the surgery,' she continued.

'Me?'

'Well, yeah, if it all goes wrong, you can still amputate it, but you may as well have a go?'

The very idea sounded ridiculous. The dreaded imposter syndrome had stopped me from even considering whether I could fix Nala's fracture myself. But what Kym said had made me think: if I could get my hands on the equipment, *could* I fix her leg?

Within veterinary practice these days, we are spoilt by the number of referral centres that have sprung up around the country, vets that have specialised in one area of veterinary medicine and are able to offer a specialist service within that field. While this makes for a brilliant service for owners and their pets, it does also create a hole in the net. What happens when owners can't afford referral, whether out of their own pockets or because their insurance won't cover it? As a GP vet, this is where we often have to make some difficult decisions and either opt for palliative care or do our best. And often, if that is something surgical, it can even mean learning while 'on the job'. This would only ever be considered with full transparency to the pet owner, though, and would often require signed consent to show understanding.

I emailed our orthopaedic surgeon. His response was encouraging. He kindly talked me through a step-by-step guide on how to place a dynamic compression plate to a type-one open forelimb fracture. I then phoned a veterinary instruments company, who also kindly offered to courier out all the various bits and pieces needed to fit a Meccano-inspired metal plate onto a dog's fractured leg. The company ran training courses on fracture repair and could spare one of the kits they use for the next week or so. They even forwarded a link to some of their online video tutorials on how to repair the fracture. There wasn't really any excuse not to at least have a go. After all, there was no owner to navigate if the surgery went wrong. Just the added expense to my boss and the sinking feeling of being a crap vet to contend with.

And so, having spent that evening scrolling through count-less online video tutorials and reading every orthopaedic textbook I could find, the following day I found myself scrubbing and prepping for Nala's surgery. I plunged the syringe of white propofol through the cannula in Nala's vein, and watched as her body relinquished consciousness to the effects of the anaesthetic drugs. We clipped the fur off her leg from her foot to her shoulder and cleaned her skin with an iodine solution the colour of a weak cup of tea. Her leg was suspended, raised high above her body and tied with a rope to a drip stand to help fatigue and stretch the muscles that had contracted around the fracture site, and then we moved her through to the operating theatre.

As I scrubbed my hands with the antiseptic solution, then clambered into an oversized surgeon's sterile gown, I could feel the beads of sweat form under my scrub cap. My glasses steamed with the flow of nervous exhaled breath as it passed from behind my surgeon's mask and escaped the wire crimp over the bridge of my nose. I placed a pale blue paper sterile gown over her body and then released the leg from its stand. The leg above the fracture site was firmly attached to her shoulder; the foot on the other hand was flapping, left to right in a plane that correlated to the fracture site.

'Well, here goes,' I said to Sarah the nurse, who was in primary control of the anaesthetic. 'Are you ready?' I asked, to which Sarah looked at me with the stethoscope in her ears and gave a confident nod.

'You've got this!' she said. The voice of encouragement and support from a veterinary nurse at times like these really does make all the difference.

With the scalpel in my hand, I made my incision over the leg. I took a pair of scissors and my forceps to start exploring down through the thin straps of muscle and eventually located the radius bone. I scraped away the muscle attachments, as Dominic, the orthopaedic surgeon, had instructed. His voice swirled in my mind, and I had printed his step-by-step email instructions onto an A4 sheet of paper and sellotaped it to the wall in theatre as a reference guide.

The first challenge would be to reduce the fracture – to try to realign the two ends of bone that had snapped in half and contracted over each other thanks to the pull of muscle attachment, making the leg look a good inch shorter than it should be. I attached two forceps to the bone – one to either side of the fracture site to allow some 'grip'. Then came the gruesome part: I tried to pull the two ends away from each other, but they would not budge. I tried again, and again, but there was not enough movement. Surely I couldn't fail at the first hurdle? Dominic had warned me that because the fracture was already a good few days old, possibly longer as we had no clue when it had actually happened, reducing the fracture would probably be the hardest part of the surgery. And he wasn't wrong.

I looked at Sarah. 'I can't bloody do it,' I said, through gritted teeth.

'Just go for it!' she replied, giving me the permission I needed to hear to put a bit of brute force into it.

I leant my body over Nala's leg and with my two elbows pulling away from each other, the same way as if I were pulling a Christmas cracker on my own, I yanked hard on both forceps. I made a grunting sound and then suddenly, by applying a slight angle, the two ends of the broken bone moved just enough that I could tilt the ends over each other as they slotted back into place.

Relief.

'Thank God for that! OK, step one done!' I looked up at Dominic's printed email on the wall. 'What's next?'

I took hold of the plate – a rectangular, flat piece of metal with numerous holes along it – and lined it up against the fracture. Using a guide, I drilled holes into Nala's bone, measured the depth, picked the right size screw and drove it through the plate, anchoring it into her bone. I worked my way along the plate – methodically drilling, guiding, measuring and screwing it in place. I got into a rhythm while Sarah continually monitored the anaesthetic. Once I was happy that the plate looked secure, I folded the muscle belly back into alignment, flushed the site with some sterile saline and sutured the skin over the metal plate.

'See,' Sarah said with a wide grin. 'Easy!'

'For you to say!' I laughed, and pointed at the copious amounts of sweat that had soaked through my scrub cap. We both chuckled together, relieved that the surgery had seemed to go relatively well.

'Let's get a quick X-ray,' I said, positioning Nala's leg as we took a post-operative radiograph.

The black and white image slowly appeared on the screen. It wasn't quite perfect – two of the screws were perhaps a little too generous for the size of the bone – but overall it didn't look half bad. The leg was, at least, back in alignment, and furthermore, it was still attached to Nala's body. It was a good start, surely? Sarah spun the dial on the anaesthetic machine to switch off the sevoflurane anaesthetic gas, then she squeezed the black rubber bag attached to the pipework on the anaesthetic machine to flush clean oxygen through to Nala's lungs and allow her to start waking up.

I pulled the gown off and swept the surgeon's cap from

my head, my hair flattened with perspiration as though I'd been in a racing car with my head stuck out of the window. Then as I pulled the mask from over my face and let it hang around my neck, the first breath of fresh air flowed freely into my lungs as I realised I'd done it. The plate was in, the fracture was fixed, Nala had survived her painful orthopaedic operation and I could go back to finishing up the rest of the morning consultations.

For me, the day had only just started, but for Nala there lay ahead six long weeks of rest and recuperation to allow her leg to heal. But I couldn't leave Nala in the surgery for six weeks, so that evening I loaded up some syringes of pain relief and she came home to live with Mark, Oliver and me. We set up a temporary kennel in the kitchen to restrict her movements, I continued her analgesia overnight and she slept quietly next to Oliver. In the day she came to work with me, where she had Oliver for company as she stayed in the kennel (as part of her continued post-operative care). Gradually we started some basic training and over the few weeks I grew more and more fond of having her in our home. She came back to Yorkshire with me that Christmas and met both sides of our family. She followed Oliver around wherever he went, but thanks to the cumbersome dressing on her left leg, had to spend most of her time in the crate. But without a doubt, she was a complete and utter joy. And not once did she lose her zest or love for being in the company of humans.

The first rule of being a vet is having the self-discipline to not take your 'work' home! It's also the first rule most vets break at some point in their careers! But sadly at the time we just weren't in the right pace to take on a second dog long term. I knew from the day I brought her home I would only foster Nala until I could find her a suitable forever home. And luckily that day soon arrived and I found Nala the most incredible family who adored her as much as I did. With time she went on to make a full recovery.

I still see Nala. She lives a beautiful life and is able to enjoy all the spoils that come with a loving family. And every time I see her, her reaction is still the same: her tail starts to wag, her bottom wiggles from side to side and she licks and licks and licks. I'm sure she knows.

After such a rough beginning, to have played a part in Nala's transformation and success story will always be a true highlight of my career. And I don't mean in a 'pat my own back' kind of way, but more as a reflection of our entire profession: from my boss at the time, who facilitated her treatment without question, to the nurses who took Nala under their wings and into their hearts; the receptionists who supported the team from out front, to the orthopaedic surgeon who found time in his own busy schedule to guide me through the surgery without making me feel inept, and the instrument supply company who lent me their kit; to Mark and Oliver for sheltering Nala through her recovery; and finally her forever family who came forward and offered her the happy ending she truly deserved. At every stage it was a team effort, and one I will always be proud to have been part of.

CHAPTER 13

Barney

'I'd like t'give 'im a fair chance,' she said, in her familiar West Yorkshire accent. Then with her two hands pressed into a prayer position, she rocked them backwards and forwards over the small plastic pet carrier cage, as she slowly spoke the words, 'but I jus' think, at the end o'day, I'd like to treat 'im for the animal that he is.' She clenched her two fists together and continued. 'I don't want to think of 'im in any pain, so I will tek the painkillers, but . . . when t'time's right . . . I'll bring 'im back and we can do as necessary so he d'unt 'av to suffer.' She lowered her hands, indicating that her beautifully articulate, succinct verdict was final and this was the treatment option she was most comfortable with.

We had spent the past twenty minutes or so discussing the options around what, if anything, we should do with the new pea-sized mass that had erupted out of nowhere on the flank of her beloved pet rat. It was actually her teenage son's rat, but Sammy (the rat) had become an even bigger part of her son's life since his father walked out on them a few months previously.

'He'll be absolutely devastated,' she shared with me, when I said there was a very high chance the mass would be cancerous. But Sammy was already three and a half years old, a good age for a rat, and I had already surgically removed two masses under general anaesthetic in the preceding six months. 'Where d'yer draw the line?' was her fair reaction. 'If we lost 'im under t'anaesthetic when he could've otherwise just lived on comfortable for a few more months, we'd be gutted.'

We both agreed. Ultimately it would be her son's decision, she said, but she thanked for me for taking the time to go through the options. It's often the case with smaller pets. Owners can feel either judged for getting emotional over a gerbil or a hamster or as if there's nothing we can offer except to suggest putting them to sleep. Actually, often (especially now) there is a lot we can do for the 'small furries', as they're affectionately referred to among vets. But there is still often a tendency to ridicule the significance and importance of these smaller pets. 'A rat? Why would someone spend money on a rat?' I've heard many an opinionated voice uttered from those on the outside looking in. But the reality is, the value of a pet's life is not based on the size, species, breed, or the price tag they carried at the time of 'purchase'. It is something far more nuanced than that. I have seen grown adults cry over lost guinea pigs. Pet chickens that have been willingly referred to an avian specialist vet. And many thousands of pounds spent on a rabbit with slowed gut motility. And who are any of us to judge? The bond owners feel with their pets is real, regardless of the species.

After two months on pain relief, Sammy's lump had inevitably grown as predicted. He'd started to gnaw at it and the skin had ulcerated. There was a slight smell developing, despite their best efforts to keep bathing the scab with salt water. Eventually the time had come for him to be put to sleep. The son accompanied his mother. Perhaps fifteen years old, arguably a particularly difficult stage in life for men to express or understand their emotions. Through bloodshot eyes, he reluctantly handed Sammy over to me. His mother placed an arm around his shoulders, giving him enough distance and independence not to feel smothered, but enough of an invitation to cry on her shoulders if he needed to. He gave Sammy a kiss on the nose then hovered his cupped palms in front of him as he gradually separated them, allowing Sammy to gently fall through the gap into my hands.

'Don't worry, he'll not bite yer,' he said, as a small tear fell from his eyes. I thanked him and said what a brilliant job he'd done looking after Sammy, that he was making the kindest decision in putting his pet's needs first. He nodded and continued to cry. His mother stood behind her son, looked at me and mouthed a silent 'thank you'. He turned and, without embarrassment, hugged his mother, the way a toddler might after they've fallen, as I carried Sammy out of the consult room.

Moments like these make the job so incredibly bittersweet at times. I don't enjoy these days. Who would? Witnessing a young person lose their companion and emotional support while already going through a turbulent time felt hugely unfair. But my duty as a vet is to protect and preserve animal welfare. And I had had to learn quickly that, however experienced you are, you can't fix everyone or everything. From an animal welfare perspective, it was absolutely the best course of action.

Furthermore, I had a waiting room full of patients to get through, and my next consult was a family who had brought their new kitten in for a first vaccination. There's figuratively and literally no time allowed for melancholy while working as a vet. Like an actor flipping between the scenes of a play, as my sad face frowned through one consult, it had to transform into a jubilant smile for the next.

As a vet, euthanasia is always the great elephant in the room. I often think how strange it is that as a vet, one part of my job is to offer 'death' as a paid service. Death, as a topic, is something we just don't talk about in Western cultures. It is shrouded with mystery, sadness and hurt. But as a vet I learnt very early on that I would have to get comfortable discussing death – cosy up to it, shake hands with it, dice with it, trick it, sometimes give in to it. Other times choose it. When death is offered as a choice – an elective decision – it can also bring great comfort, relief, maybe even gratitude sometimes.

When you qualify as a vet, and get released into practice, there's a first time for absolutely everything. The first time you select which antibiotic to prescribe, the first injection, the first diagnosis, the first anaesthetic, the first surgery and, of course, the first euthanasia consultation. As students, euthanasia was the one area we didn't really get very much direct exposure or experience in. It would be entirely inappropriate to have a vet student in the corner of a room, watching on and observing a family say their final goodbyes while making notes. Often, the vet in charge would ask the student to 'sit this one out' – understandable. However, for the vet student, this renders the euthanasia consult an enigma, a mystery. We had done some rather awkward role play at uni with actors, but, to all intents and purposes, the first euthanasia consult was essentially a baptism of fire – have everything ready prepared and *just don't screw it up.*

They say you never forget your first euthanasia. For me, that's very true. Although my first experience of euthanasia came far sooner than I had ever imagined.

As we broke for the first Easter break of the first year of vet school, still wet behind the ears and with a belly full of butterflies, I left our halls of residence, packed my rickety Vauxhall Corsa and travelled to my very first farm placement – three weeks of lambing on a large country estate in East Cumbria. The farm manager, David, was a true man of the land and expected hard work. I stayed with an older couple. I liked them. I can remember thinking how extraordinarily happy they both seemed in each other's company. They shared jokes and muttered to each with their mutually unique sense of humour. It was as though Mr Kipling had met Aunt Bessie and they had both lived happily ever after.

I shared a small bedroom with another guy called Alex who was only in his early thirties but looked at least a decade older. He had been drafted in as a 'relief lamber', a self-employed shepherd from Dorset who moved from temporary contract to temporary contract across various farms, picking up the extra work required around lambing time. He was good to have around, and to learn from. Seasoned. Knowledgeable. Patient.

David, not one to give up easily on his flock, believed even the sickest of lambs should at least be given a chance and so

every few hours, through day or night, we donned impermeable gloves and gowns (a biosecurity measure to reduce the
risk of disease transmission) and fed a group of little lambs
via a stomach tube as they wouldn't (or rather couldn't)
suckle naturally. We cleaned the diarrhoea from their
hindquarters with warm water and cotton wool and then
smothered them with Vaseline to stop the liquid faeces from
burning their skin. Unfortunately, despite our best efforts,
the prognosis was looking more and more bleak as the time
ticked by.

That morning I was on mucking out duty. From across the
barn, I had caught a glimpse of David and Alex in discussion
by the kitchen. Too far away for me to hear their conversation, I could see they were both nodding in agreement on
something. David left the barn, and I could see from the
corner of my eye Alex walking over towards me. He picked
up a fork and began to compress the top layer of soiled straw
bedding to fit another forkful in the barrow before wheeling
it to the muck heap.

While doing so, he started talking. 'One of the sick lambs
has gone downhill overnight,' he said, as I continued to heave
another forkful of straw over the fence. 'David's said to let
it go.'

After all our efforts and the collective hours we had invested, it was hard not to feel a little disappointed to be
throwing in the towel. Although I had already started to
question in my own mind how fair it was for us to keep going.
And so, feeling deflated but aware that we were losing the
battle, and not wanting to watch the poor lamb suffer unnec-
essarily, I nodded in agreement.

'He's asked if you wanna do it?' Alex asked casually, as he

heaved another weighty fork of used straw bedding over the side of the pen and into the wheelbarrow.

'Me?' I replied, as I pointed my own finger to my chest and felt my heart quicken. It was as though I had just been singled out at school, picked to play a sport for which I didn't understand the rules. His words caught me completely off guard. And they hit me like a train. Whether it was the way he asked so bluntly, so casually, or just that feeling of being woefully inadequate to complete the task required of me, I stood in silence for a moment, simply staring at him.

I was unsure how to answer and worried there had been some sort of misunderstanding. Perhaps the two men thought I was further into my veterinary training than I was. I could take that as a compliment, being only a few months in. But no, I'd rather have kept my student ego in check and rectify their mistake. I followed up with a, 'Well, I've . . . err . . . I've never actually put anything to sleep.'

'Really?' Alex said, surprised. 'Well, I'm happy to walk you through it, but it's up to you.'

It may sound surprising, but euthanasia is not actually classed as an act of veterinary surgery and so by law, it can be carried out by anyone. It doesn't have to be a vet. But legally it does have to be humane. And painless. However, being closer to having finished sixth-form college than I was to finishing my veterinary degree, I had assumed we would build up to this day much more slowly; that it would be somehow protected under a veterinary 'rite of passage', that we would be mentored until authorised to carry out such a hugely important act. At the time, I didn't have any first-hand experience of euthanasia. We'd had some very brief lectures on the humane dispatch of farm animals – a black and white diagram of a cow's head, with dotted lines drawn at angles to each other between the eyes and ears to form an 'X' on the forehead. I had a vague understanding of the theory but to actually put that knowledge into practice felt like a very different ball game. And yet, there I was, thrown in at the deep end only a few months into my first ever placement.

But Alex and I had developed a good working relationship. I trusted him, we'd helped each other out and I knew he was a good teacher. And so, on the understanding it was with David's blessing, I tentatively agreed. We propped our forks up against the wheelbarrow and walked over to the hospital pen. As we walked, Alex explained in detail how things should happen. He had picked up a black plastic briefcase that David had left by the kitchen and as we reached the edge of the pen, he lay the case on the floor, released the two metal latches and opened it to reveal a handgun. Outlined and protected by a foam casing, Alex carefully picked up the gun, then handed it over to me. Not actually a gun that fires bullets, instead a captive bolt hand pistol that fires a retractable cylindrical bolt (like a 'bottle cork') to stun an animal, rendering them immediately unconscious.

I'd never held a gun before. I don't think I had even seen that many guns in my life other than in museums or on television. To be in the presence of a weapon, and then to hold that weapon in my hand, made everything suddenly feel very serious. Dangerous, even. The cold, metal pistol was surprisingly heavy in my hand. It demanded respect. I felt the weight of the weapon hang by my side. Alex continued to arrange the set, as though preparing a scene for a stage show.

Frail and unable to lift the weight of its own head, the lamb seemed to be drifting in and out of consciousness under the warm red glow of the heat lamp. Alex leant over the pen and retrieved the weakened lamb, which dangled in his hands like a stuffed child's toy. He lowered him down in a pile of clean straw. In a desperate reflex reaction of fight or flight, the weakened lamb shuddered and pushed a front leg out in front of the other in an attempt to stand. Unable, though, he collapsed under his own weight and fell face forwards into the straw. Alex caught him just in time, and slowly lowered him into a steady, comfortable position.

Standing by my side, he then explained the procedure once again. I listened intently to his words – the rules, the aim, the commitment, the firm grip, the steady arm, the one chance to 'get it right'. The pressure felt enormous. I was trembling. My clammy hand made the ice-cold metal of the pistol feel slippery. I placed my free hand on the other side of the firearm to steady the grip and hovered the end of the pistol towards the lamb. With the tip of the gun occupying what seemed to be the whole surface area of the tiny lamb's forehead, I checked my aim, held my breath and then on a silent count of three in my head, stroked my index finger into the curved arc and pulled the trigger.

The bang from the pistol reverberated around the shed. The sound echoed for what felt like an eternity – an immediate and everlasting reminder of what had just happened, what I had done, hammering it into my brain over and over again that for the first time ever, I had just purposefully ended another animal's life. The lamb lay motionless. Alex took a knife from his pocket and finally the lamb looked at peace.

'That was really well done, mate,' Alex said quietly, while looking up at me. 'I actually didn't think you'd do it!' He stood up, took the gun from my hand, untucked the front panel of his shirt from his trouser waist and used a clean patch of fabric to wipe the blood from the metal tip. 'The first one is always the hardest, but you did that really well.'

I felt numb. As we packed everything away, those feelings melted into a strange mix of sadness and relief. I was relieved that the lamb was no longer suffering, sad because it had to happen (and it did *have* to happen) but mostly grateful that it was all over so quickly. I also remember feeling bizarrely quite proud of myself, that Alex said I had done a 'good job'. That might sound boastful, but it wasn't pride in a 'puffed chest' way, but rather a quiet self-respect that I *had* managed to go through with it and that I *had* prevented an animal from suffering with a clean, painless and humane death. It was my first glimpse of what it felt like to be a real vet with real responsibilities. You never forget the first euthanasia.

That was then, but after graduating as a vet, the responsibility of respecting death is the one constant that never changes. The discussion, the emotion, the weight of responsibility never dwindles; it never gets easier. It perhaps gets more 'streamlined', but it still feels just as important to 'get it right' every single time now as it did for the very first time.

There are times, though, when I am so very thankful that I have the ability and licence to perform rapid, humane euthanasia. Those rare times when I am up against something so excruciatingly upsetting that I will actively hurry, as fast as I possibly can, to relieve an animal's suffering, and worry about the 'whys' and 'how comes' after. As was the case on my first Boxing Day out-of-hours shift, having been called to a yearling foal just after 7 a.m. A stunning morning – crisp and cold, the hilltop lanes were barely passable. Underfoot, the frosted tarmac snaked through a picture-perfect white wonderland. The beautiful, dappled grey foal frolicked in the white, frosty paddock, turned out from his stable to experience snow for the first time as his young owner, filled with excitement, hoped to capture the joyful moment on their camera.

The ground glistened as the golden sun continued to rise, the yellow light bathing the yearling foal as I scrambled on the frozen ground to access his jugular vein. I connected the syringe as quickly as I could and helped him drift, peacefully but rapidly, towards his final breath. His eyes glazed over as he lay, tangled in the invisible, lethal boundary that he had galloped straight through at full speed. The pool of red snow on the ground around him acted as a timely reminder of the significant dangers that silently lurk along any horse paddock encircled with barbed-wire fencing.

Most people, when I tell them I am a vet, say that it must be the worst part of the job – putting an animal to sleep. The truth is, though, strangely, it's not.

Yes, it can be upsetting, traumatic even, but every animal I have ever euthanised has been for a purpose, and that purpose is always because it is in the best interests of that animal at that time. Of course, it is never going to be a 'perk' of the job, but there is something poignant and perhaps reassuring to know I have prevented an animal from suffering.

Barney was a beautiful golden retriever. He had a big square head, a large brown nose shaped like a bear and black circles around both of his eyes that made him look as though he was wearing some perfectly applied eyeliner. I'd met him and his owner a couple of times, but I wouldn't say I knew them that well – not at the start anyway. He was kind, gentle, and would happily plod into my consult room with his hairy tail perched at half mast, like pampas grass swaying in a gentle sea breeze.

But, at eight years old, he had developed a strange 'tiredness' about him, and had perhaps gained a little weight. His owner, Mel, had put it down to him getting older, but that morning he had collapsed in the garden and had been unable to stand up.

They arrived as an emergency and I had been the vet to see them in. I met them in the car park, and Barney was in the boot of their estate car. He had his head raised, he was conscious, but even on first glance I could see he was short of breath. His body rocked forwards and backwards with each panting breath, the front part of his abdomen sinking in and out, alternating with his chest movements, suggesting he was having to engage his abdominal muscles in order to fill his chest cavity with air.

'He, he just fell . . . dropped down, then couldn't get back up,' Mel said, wiping her nose with a tissue. 'My God, it scared the life out of me. I thought he'd died,' she said, tears welling in her eyes.

We carried Barney through into the practice and lay him on a few piled-up dog beds put out by the nursing team in my consulting room. His abdomen was swollen. Mel had noticed the change in shape but thought he was perhaps just putting on weight. With my hands, though, I could sense the rounded shape felt more like a water balloon, swishing and swirling around. 'Ascites' is the term to indicate a free fluid build-up in the abdominal cavity – it can link to a whole myriad of conditions, from protein changes within the blood, to infectious causes, cancerous causes or even a number of heart conditions that can alter the various pressures along the body's circulatory system, leading to the condition termed 'right-sided heart failure'.

I attempted to palpate the abdomen, but being so swollen, it was impossible to differentiate any particular structures. By this point, Barney was lying on his front with his head rested gently between his two front paws, quietly observing the kerfuffle around him and still managing to offer up the occasional tail wag each time I gave his head a stroke.

I tucked my stethoscope under his left elbow and listened over his ribcage. Normally, for a dog of his size, I'd expect the heart to be easily audible. But with Barney, I couldn't pick up any heart sounds at all. I moved the drum of the stethoscope forwards a centimetre, then back. I moved over to the right side of his chest, but still no sounds. *This is ridiculous*, I thought to myself, *he's alive so there must be a heartbeat!*

I returned to the left side of his chest, adjusted the rubber seal in both my ears, leant forwards and indicated politely to Mel that I'd need a couple of minutes' complete silence to listen carefully to his heart. Then, with the room silent, I could just hear the faintest thudding sound of his heart. Not the usual *'lub dub'* sound you might expect, but rather, an erratic plethora of thumping sounds, like a pair of trainers randomly beating against the drum as they spin through a washing machine cycle.

'It's looking like this could be something cardiac,' I summarised, 'that has caused a build-up of fluid in his abdomen, possibly also his chest, but I can't say for sure whether the changes in his heart are the primary cause or they are as a result of something else.'

Mel listened intently, taking in every word.

'Of course, there are options – but if you're keen for me to try and work out more, then I think we need to take some chest X-rays, run some blood work and perform an ultrasound examination of his heart.'

She was keen. After such an abrupt shock, she didn't want to say goodbye there and then, and if there was any hope of saving him, she wanted to explore all avenues.

Barney stayed with us for the day. I placed the ultrasound probe against his chest wall. The heart chambers were contracting and dilating. The heart muscle looked a normal thickness. However, there was a large black shadow circling around the outline of Barney's heart. This blackened perimeter around the paler grey appearance of his heart wall could indicate only one thing: fluid. Fluid that shouldn't be there. Fluid around the heart, trapped in a sack known as the pericardium. The heart was essentially bobbing around like champagne cork in a pint of water and could no longer fill or contract efficiently. It explained why the heart was so quiet, in the same way the sound travelling underwater is muffled. Fluid had also accumulated in his abdomen, which accounted for the supposed 'weight gain'. The poor lad had become exhausted. However, worryingly, there was more. I then spotted something else that shouldn't be there. Sitting just next to his right atrium, a grey egg-shaped structure, not recognisable within a normal heart. An uninvited guest, a gate crasher to the party. The 'egg' was something known as a 'heart base tumour'. Barney had cancer of the heart.

We discussed the options, and Mel was keen for me to perform pericardiocentesis to drain the excess fluid around his heart and help to alleviate the immediate pressure – draining fluid around the heart is not without risks, even the sedation alone is high risk due to the cardiac compromise, but there was no other option if we were to save his life.

With Barney lying still, the nurses clipped and surgically prepared his chest wall. I counted along the ridges of his thorax to identify the sixth rib space and injected some local anaesthetic. Using a scalpel blade, I made a small stab incision through the skin, then took hold of the stylet and, with a firm push through the chest wall, felt the catheter 'pop' through the pericardial sac into the fluid bath surrounding the heart. I removed the metal stylet and advanced the soft rubber tube, keeping an eye on the ECG reading and ensuring I had not accidentally popped into the heart muscle itself. Always a tense moment. I began to withdraw on the syringe and drained an extraordinary half litre of bloody, watery fluid from the space around Barney's heart. We sent samples off for analysis, but with the presence of the tumour, it was already apparent what the root cause of the fluid build-up was.

Remarkably, the heart can immediately function near normally again after the procedure, and after a couple of days, Barney's demeanour had improved entirely. His swollen abdomen had begun to deflate, his breathing rate and effort relaxed and he was almost back to being his normal self. His quality of life was arguably excellent. We talked through the option to take him for specialist surgery – heart surgery through the chest wall to attempt to reduce the tumour size and cut a window through the pericardial sac itself. They concluded that wasn't the right option for them and so instead we periodically drained the fluid as his signs (inevitably) recurred every few months.

Several months after the initial diagnosis, and after three

separate procedures to drain the fluid, the tumour on his heart had doubled in size. On the final drain, it only bought a few days of relief before the signs of tiredness, exhaustion and heavy breathing crept back in. By this point, I had grown to know the family very well – Mel, her husband and their two daughters, both in their mid twenties, who I'd also met on several occasions. We had spent many hours discussing the pros and cons of all the options, reviewing and re-reviewing things at each step. After each consult, Mel would thank me, reach her hand out and gently place her fingertips on the side of my face – 'Thank you, thank you for everything you're doing for us. And for Barney.'

When the decision came to relieve Barney of any further interventions, to allow him a dignified and peaceful end, to stop all treatment and let him finally be at rest, the family had asked if I might drive to their house so he could pass away at home, on his bed in front of the fire. It is a very personal decision, whether to opt for euthanasia on neutral ground – such as the vet's – and leave memories of that painful day with us, or whether to perform it within the home. There is no right or wrong. Barney and his family felt more comforted by the idea of Barney passing away peacefully at home.

We gathered around, I made the necessary preparations, counselled the family through what to expect and, as they said their goodbyes, Barney lay his head between his two huge front paws. I administered the injection and he drifted off peacefully towards his final sleep.

I am normally very good at detaching myself from my work. I have to be. But with Barney, I let myself get closer than normal. We cried together. I don't regret that at all. The family were so kind and having spent months looking after him, the affection they showed him was catching. On some level, through their love for him, I think I started to love him as my own as well. Some might say that I grew too attached. So be it. But the words Mel wrote in the thank-you card they sent me exuded such kindness, such gratitude – and included the most beautiful tribute to Barney – that above all I feel honoured to have been able to help such a kind, loving family through their time of sorrow as they said their final goodbyes to their most treasured Barney.

Euthanasia may seem like the worst part of my job, but it isn't. I consider it a privilege to share in these moments. What many people perhaps don't realise is that whenever I put an animal to sleep, despite the upset and the sadness, it is often at that very moment when you can most feel the abundance of love in the room. The love people have for their pets shines so brightly in these selfless moments of kindness. And that is what I remember most about Barney. Losing a pet is unbearably sad, and I don't think it ever gets any easier, but the one thing I have learnt about saying goodbye is that the sadness we feel on losing them is a reflection of the love we have for them in our hearts. And with that, you could say nothing loved is ever lost.

CHAPTER 14

Oliver, Part III

I hurried my car through the gates and into the car park, opened the boot and heaved Oliver up towards my chest. His body was heavy. I pivoted backwards with my hips to help take some of the strain from the almost forty-kilogram weight in my arms, then stumbled step by step into the practice. *Don't trip, don't trip, DON'T TRIP*, is all I could keep saying to myself, as I navigated the small staircase past reception with Oliver in my arms. It was just past eight o'clock in the morning, the busy rush of patients and appointments hadn't quite started, although at that point Oliver was my only priority. The rest of my veterinary colleagues had also only just arrived to start their day, hanging their coats, hiding in the consult room to swiftly change into their scrubs and then flicking on the kettle to start the first of many caffeine hits to help get us all through the busy schedule of appointments.

With Oliver in my arms, I turned and pushed my back through the double swinging doors that led to the prep area. They made a loud bang against the wall as I entered. I lowered

FOR THE LOVE OF ANIMALS

Oliver onto the prep room table and the nursing team immediately dropped whichever routine task they'd been assigned and assembled around him like a well-rehearsed group of superheroes.

'He's been hit by a car,' I said calmly.

Then, surrounded by the familiarity of my own work environment, I slipped into vet mode. My head was racing at a million miles an hour as I tried to decipher how I should tackle things clinically, the steps I needed to take to effectively triage my 'patient' and prioritise each intervention. I knew that if I stood any chance of saving his life, I'd have to think on my feet. Stay rational, be efficient, keep calm and think methodically. For a split second, I was able to disassociate from Oliver being my own dog and instead consider him as a walk-in emergency. I had no choice but to switch off. I had to pretend that I had just arrived at work, and it was somebody else's dog that had just been rushed through the prep room doors.

'Can we get some oxygen, please,' I called to the team. 'And let's get an IV line into him.'

But, as I looked up, I could see the nursing team had already assembled the anaesthetic machine. A clear plastic conical-shaped mask had been placed over Oliver's nose – the rubber diaphragm created a seal around his muzzle to help guide the steady flow of oxygenated air into his lungs. Another nurse had already lined up a cannula with tape and bandages and was clipping a small patch of fur from his hind leg to gain intravenous access. A drip stand had a clear plastic one-litre bag of Hartmann's intravenous fluid hanging from it, with a giving set primed and ready to connect to the end of the cannula. And behind me another nurse had already retrieved the small brown glass bottle of methadone from the locked safe and was drawing up the correct dose of soothing opiate pain relief that Oliver so desperately needed. Veterinary nurses *are* superheroes.

At that point, the head nurse also walked into the prep room and came straight over to me. 'Are you OK?' she asked.

It was only then that I felt myself unable to carry on 'acting' as the vet. 'No,' I replied. Since receiving the awful phone call, I had managed to remain with it. I'd kept it together and felt like I had lived up to the enormous pressure to take lead as 'the vet' in the family. But in that moment, in my workplace surrounded by my colleagues, I metaphorically stepped onto the other side of my consulting-room table. As our skilled nursing team took over, I finally felt permitted to swap from being the vet in charge to just being Oliver's dad. And through that moment I allowed myself to feel the same worry, concern, grief and guilt that I'd seen so many other pet owners experience in my consulting room. And *that* was the moment I broke.

Through unimaginable worry, tears welled in my eyes and streamed down my face. 'I just feel so guilty,' I said to our head nurse as she hugged me close.

My nostrils streamed with mucus as though I'd been struck down with a nasty bout of flu. Basic words half rolled and half flopped off my tongue – there was no chance that I could form an *actual* sentence. And any of the gulping throat sounds that did manage to escape through my vocal cords made me sound like an asphyxiated toad. Once I start, I have a knack of throwing myself absolutely headfirst into that deeply unattractive, ugly phase of crying: bloodshot eyes, snot everywhere, my whole body doing weird jerky movements and then normally, at some point, I'll snort. The floodgates of emotion had opened, and our poor head nurse found herself at eight o'clock in the morning having to wrap her arms around the vet that was, in less than thirty minutes, supposed to start consulting.

The nurses rattled off a few X-rays while I stood in the kitchen being consoled by my boss, who quickly realised her inflamed, mucus-leaching, beetroot-red, crying vet could no way step out into the public domain. And so kindly, I was offered the day off to focus on Oliver.

'James, do you want to come and have a look at these?' Kym the nurse called from the darkened X-ray room.

With Oliver lying comfortably on his side, snoozing under the hefty influence of his recent hit of methadone, the black and white radiograph images of his insides filled the computer screen. I wiped the tears, snot and mucus from my face and assessed the pictures in front of me. Chest intact. Good. Diaphragm intact. Bladder intact. Pelvis intact. Both back legs intact. This was all good news. Left front leg intact. Then right front leg – not intact.

Not even close to being intact.

'Bloody hell, it looks like someone's taken a sledgehammer to him,' I summarised. 'Let's set up the scanner.'

An ultrasound scan of Oliver's abdomen showed there was no free fluid, no blood. His spleen looked normal; his bladder was still round. Everything looked as it should. This was also good.

The image of Oliver running into the road, playing joyfully, unaware of the oncoming danger about to hit his blind side, filled my mind. A surge of hurt filled my heart as my eyes welled once again. Although this was soon followed by an even bigger surge of pet owner guilt. How could I have been so stupid to not lock the front door? If I had just dropped the latch, the door would never have opened, no matter how many times the two rascal canine teenagers jumped at it, and *none* of this would have happened.

Oliver gave a slow attempt to lift his head. 'Hey, buddy!' I said to him, as though he would somehow answer back, an example of the great conundrum: why *do* we talk to our pets? 'How you feeling?' I asked, again inexplicably.

I stroked over his head and down his two soft ears. His tongue lolled out of his mouth in the gap that had been created by his offset jaw from the trauma as a puppy. I could always tell when he had fallen into a really, *really* deep sleep at home when his tongue lolled. I was besotted with how adorable it looked. I used to film it on my phone or take a quick photograph while he was sleeping. I often think, if our pets *could* talk, how horrified they'd be to discover the thousands of photos of themselves on our mobile phones; pictures *and videos* of them sleeping, eating, playing, travelling in the car, on holiday, on walks, on the beach, even in the bath. With Kym's help, I moved Oliver through to a kennel the nurses had arranged for him. A deep bed lay over a heat mat to help keep him warm after the recent ordeal. While he was still snoozing, Kym placed a thick multi-layered bandage, known as a 'Robert Jones' dressing, over Oliver's leg to stabilise the fracture, and I left them to make a phone call.

With Oliver's leg shattered into pieces, it was immediately apparent that fixing it would be beyond my clinical level of expertise. And so later that afternoon, I found myself transferring Oliver back into the boot of my car and heading up the motorway to our nearest veterinary referral hospital. I'd referred countless cases to Dominic over the years, we had spoken on both the phone and via email, but we'd never actually met in person. I pulled up in *their* car park and walked into *their* reception area. This was unfamiliar territory. I'd crossed the threshold into another vet's practice. The smell was familiar, but the phones had a different ringtone, the receptionists wore a different uniform – and headsets. It felt somehow familiar, but not quite home.

'Hi, I'm here with Oliver,' I said to the lady behind reception. 'I spoke with Dominic earlier.'

'Oh yes, do you want to bring him in? Dom's expecting you so you can go straight through.'

I returned to the car once again to heave my heavy lump of broken Labrador into another veterinary building. This time for specialist orthopaedic surgery. Dominic called me through to the consulting room and I lay Oliver on the piece of vet bed that had been laid out for him. I had already sent him the radiographs, which he had pulled up on his computer that connected to a television screen on the wall – the projected image of Oliver's shattered front leg filled the screen.

'So,' Dominic started, as he took out a pen from his pocket and started making squiggly movements across the fracture site. The pen marked in a semi-circle one side of the fracture, then the other. Then he pretended to snap the pen in half, and then started making similar sweeping hand gestures down his own arm to try to explain the various forces involved in the repair of a fracture like Oliver's.

Strangely, I can remember the room, I can remember Oliver's face, I can remember Dominic – but I cannot for the life of me remember a word of what he actually said. Partly, probably, because he was using a lot of orthopaedic technical jargon and went into minute detail over which screw he might use, which plate, which suture material – weighing up the pros and cons of each. I could sense his passion. He was calm but raring to go – a surgeon is never happier than with a scalpel in his or her hand – and the specialist knowledge cascaded from him as he outlined the intricacies of his surgical plan. Maybe he had gone into extra detail, thinking he could indulge in a slightly more informed 'vet to vet' client discussion, or maybe he hadn't, I honestly couldn't tell you, for in that moment all I focused on and all I cared about was Oliver.

I signed the consent form. Handed over my insurance details. And prayed it would cover the four and a half thousand pound estimate I had just committed to spending. Sometimes people are surprised that as a vet I have insurance for my own pets. But there is absolutely no way I could have afforded Oliver's treatment without it.

I felt my eyes well up once again. I felt embarrassed to be so irrationally emotional. Even a bit ashamed that in front of my fellow veterinary professionals, I wasn't acting professional and keeping it together. I knew, on balance, that Oliver had had a lucky escape – if all he suffered was a broken leg, we could fix that, I *knew* that. Things could have been far worse. I *knew* that too. But still, the worry in my heart was immeasurable.

'Sorry, I'm so stupid!' I said under my breath and wiped the tears from my eyes before they had a chance to fall down my face. But then, I thought . . . *bollocks to it*. I leant forwards and gave Oliver a huge kiss on the top of his head. His confused face looked up at me, and with his square head gently resting in my cupped hands, I told him everything was going to be OK. I watched as Dominic, with the help of a nurse, lifted the four corners of the blanket, and on the count of three, like a wounded soldier being carried off the battlefield, they raised Oliver off the ground and slowly walked towards the door. And with that, they took him away. There was nothing more I could do.

There is one decision all vets will likely have to face at some point if they have pets of their own: whether or not you would choose to operate on your own pet? Whether you would ask someone to do it on your behalf or could perform the surgery with your own gloved hands? For some vets, it is a step too close for comfort, and there is the worry over how to stay calm and think rationally if a complication arose mid-surgery. For others, it perhaps feels too much of a burden to pass that responsibility on to a colleague. For me, on balance, I would far rather it be on my shoulders to carry the weight if (heaven forbid) something did go wrong, and so I've always felt quite instinctively that if given the choice, I'd prefer to perform surgery myself. Which made it even harder to helplessly stand back and hand Oliver over to another vet in his time of need.

I had previously taken Oliver to surgery myself back when he was only ten months old. Firstly, I had surgically removed his right mandibular canine tooth (his lower right fang) as a result of the traumatic jaw fracture he'd suffered as a youngster. His jawbone had healed but his teeth were offset and out of alignment, which meant that every time he closed his jaw his bottom right canine created a painful indentation in the roof of his mouth. The only realistic option at the time was extraction. So I cut the gum, created a flap and burred through his jawbone to perform the extraction. The canine tooth of a Labrador is surprisingly large – it looks more like a dinosaur relic, or like a whale's tooth that has been washed up on the beach. For a very brief moment I thought about drilling a hole through it, and polishing it up to wear like a surfer's necklace on some twine. But I don't surf and I didn't live anywhere near a beach, so I decided on balance that wearing my dog's extracted tooth around my neck would probably be a bit weird!

Then I had to sort his missing eye. The damaged eyeball had already been tied off and removed by the breeder at the time of the accident, but the 'socket' was still present, including the conjunctiva and all tear-producing structures, meaning a brown smear of tear-stained fur had leached from the corner of his eye socket and down his face. For this I performed an enucleation procedure, which is an operation to remove the eyeball and all the surrounding structures. I had to adapt the technique as Oliver's actual eyeball was already missing, and carefully navigate the traumatised tissue to ensure I had removed anything functional before I could finally sew his eyelid permanently closed.

And then lastly, to go in for the hat trick, I also whipped his balls off.

But this time, things were very different. His smashed-up leg was not something I could fix. It was undoubtedly beyond my clinical expertise. Referral was by far the best option. And so Oliver stayed in the hospital overnight with a plan to operate the following day.

Although I knew he was in the safest hands, sitting at home with Mark that evening, without Oliver barking, doing zoomies around the living room or his 'Tigger bounce', the house felt desperately quiet. I thought about how much he had transformed our lives in the eighteen months since we picked him up as a puppy. I was actually quite taken aback at how emotional I was to have left him in the hospital; to feel so much worry and concern over what some would say is 'just a dog'. But, as anyone knows who has loved a dog, no dog is ever 'just a dog'. I often think, maybe on some level we see our pets as a projection of ourselves. The world is a far less daunting or scary place when there is another you by your side to face it with. That was certainly the case with Oliver.

For me, it all goes back to finding my confidence about my 'real self'. Coming out, as revelationary and empowering as it may seem, doesn't automatically cancel out all the years of lived hurt. Indeed, for many years after I came out I still carried a subconscious level of internalised shame about being gay. I would self-monitor my mannerisms in public – I couldn't hold Mark's hand, for example, or publicly share affection, all out of fear. But then Oliver came along and helped to change all of that. Dogs are an immediate ice breaker, a conversation starter. I can clearly remember sitting in a coffee shop with Mark and Oliver one day, a couple next to us with their young son, maybe four or five years old. The little boy's attention kept breaking away from his gingerbread man and colouring book to look at Oliver's face. Children often see and say it as it is, and on his third stare with a huge confused frown across his face, he pulled at his mother's sleeve to tell her 'that doggy only has one eye'. We got chatting. The mother started asking about Oliver, his eye, how long we had had him, how he coped with only one eye and whether he was born like that. The father told us he had grown up with Labradors and couldn't wait to get one when their son was a little older. Then their son came round to greet Oliver. Oliver sniffed his hand, hopeful that there may be a morsel of gingerbread on offer. The little boy stroked over his head, then tried to see if he could 'help' Oliver open his closed eye. His mother pulled his hands away. 'Oooh no, don't do that!' Oliver, being the gentle soul he was, didn't bat an eyelid (no pun indented), and continued to sniff the air for any treats that may come his way. We finished our coffees and wished them well, then left.

The more frequently these small incidental interactions happened – interactions that may seem trivial when written down on paper, but showed a level of acceptance that felt ground-breaking to me at the time – the more Oliver gently pulled me out of hiding. I can remember leaving that coffee shop with a new confidence. Slowly, through moments like this, Oliver dampened my fears and showed me that I could be myself – an openly gay man, with Mark as my partner and Oliver as our family – and that everything would be OK. And with time Oliver (and Mark) helped me to unlearn all the things I had told myself about how I would be treated if anyone found out I was gay.

The truth was, almost every single person we spoke to or interacted with focused purely on how adorable Oliver was. Feeling this acceptance from strangers made me realise quite soon that being gay wasn't the 'worst hand in a game of cards'. Of course, there will always be the hateful few, but with Oliver as my bright shining protective shield, I grew in confidence and began to challenge the prejudices. Oliver taught me that there is far more love in this world than hate. He was the catalyst I needed to start properly living my life. Having the confidence to come out was the first step but it was Oliver coming into our lives that taught me how to really *live*. And be happy.

The following day, I received a phone call from Dominic around noon to say Oliver's fracture fixation was slightly more complicated than expected, but that on the whole the surgery had gone well and I could collect him mid-afternoon. I thanked him.

A few hours later I pulled into the car park and waited in reception. Then, from over my shoulder, I heard the nurse coming through the door. 'Here he is!' she said as we were reunited in the middle of the waiting area.

Oliver slowly hobbled over with his right front leg wrapped up in a bandage so thick it looked like he was balancing on a wine bottle wrapped in one of those padded cooling jackets. As he walked towards me, he clonked the big plastic lamp-shade around his head into various obstacles as he tried to nibble the bandage wrapped around his right back leg where the cannula had been placed. But despite being cocooned in all manner of veterinary medical paraphernalia, his tail wag continued to gain momentum with each step he took once he spotted who I was.

As he reached me, he nuzzled his nose into my hand and I stroked over his head. 'Hello, my handsome boy!' I kissed the bridge of his nose. His tail, by then, was spinning in huge circles like a helicopter about to take off.

'Awwwww,' the nurse said. 'He's been really good. I'll just grab his meds and then you can shoot off.'

As we waited I knelt down in reception with him, stroked over his head and suddenly felt all the emotions come flooding back again. Firstly, the guilt that had plagued my mind, and then a tremendous and overwhelming sense of gratitude. I felt so hugely appreciative of all the vets and vet nurses that had helped me through that terrible day – from Georgie, the farm vet, who had found Oliver by the road and stopped to help, to my work colleagues and my boss who showed immediate compassion and support, to Dominic who had the skills to make Oliver better.

Mark had been waiting patiently, equally concerned and eager to get Oliver home. He'd been out to buy a new squeaky toy and a puzzle feeder to keep Oliver entertained through the compulsory eight weeks of boring recovery time that lay ahead. Of course, there was never any chance of Oliver being able to work out how to actually solve the puzzle, but it was worth a try. Mark greeted us on the doorstep, holding back an excited Jenson, who was equally eager to meet up with his best mate once again and hear all about his 'news'. We had spoken with Jenson's mum Sarah by then too. She had returned the call soon after, relieved to hear the dogs were safe, and was incredibly gracious, asking after Oliver. With no hard feelings between us, both of us aware how our dogs could 'egg' each other on when they were together, I'm very grateful to say we're still friends to this day.

After climbing the couple of steps into the house, I slowly lowered Oliver onto the lounge carpet. Mark had assembled a crate beside the sofa, Oliver's confinement for the next few weeks with strict instructions from Dominic – no running, no jumping and no playing until the surgery had healed sufficiently. But with Oliver sporting a huge lampshade cone and a massive bandage over his leg, even though the crate was designed for a Great Dane, it seemed as though he would only just fit. A long road to recovery lay ahead. After the potent cocktail of drugs from his morning surgery, Oliver wobbled through the lounge, high as a kite, then flopped down into his deep-cushioned bed. Exhausted but relieved to have him back home, we both sat stroking over his soft velvet ears and rounded head as he drifted off to sleep for the afternoon.

'Do you think he'll want any tea?' Mark asked a few hours later, looking down at a still snoozing Oliver.

'I dunno,' I replied. 'Let's try.'

I left the lounge to head through to the kitchen and opened Oliver's bag of food, then sprinkled a scoop of kibble into his ceramic bowl. But as I sprinkled the biscuits I suddenly heard Mark hollering, 'NO, NO, NO! Oliver!' I ran through with the dog bowl in my hand, to find Mark hanging on to a suddenly very wakeful Oliver – his ears pricked, his one eye bright and alert and his front feet desperately trying to reach 'lift off'. The rustle of the bag and the tinkle of biscuits as they fell into his bowl had woken Oliver from his tramadol dreams and he'd sprung straight back into 'Tigger' mode.

'He started trying to bounce!' Mark cried, looking both worried but also somewhat relieved that our old Oliver was back with us. A Labrador he was through and through, and in his mind *anything* was worth attempting if there was some food on offer.

He was home. And with time, he made a full and complete recovery.

I would never wish to go through that awful day again. But while kneeling on the floor of the veterinary practice, with Oliver cradled in my arms, in that moment, I fully understood all the worry, pain, guilt, fragility, love, apprehension and appreciation that comes with being a pet owner on the other side of the veterinary consulting-room table. Despite my falterings, veterinary medicine has always been and will always be my absolute dream job. I always knew the reason I so desperately wanted to be a vet in the first place was for the love of animals. My own animals as well as other people's. And I know now that this is the reason to carry on.

I do it for the same reason I imagine every other GP vet carries on: because there will always be animals out there in need of veterinary care from this wonderful profession I am so proud to be a part of. Animals like Oliver, who mean so much to the families and individuals who love them dearly, who would go to the ends of the earth for them and would feel the exact same level of hurt as I did when they fall sick or injured. There will be animals who suffer in the worst ways, like Rudy and Nala. And animals who mean the world to their owners, like Barney. There will be mischievous cats, like Rocky. And animals suffering with cancer, like Alice. The accidentally intoxicated animals, like Bob and Jill. I do it for Beth and her litter of puppies. Even for the occasional surprise baby elephant! As vets and vet nurses, we are there for them all.

And in that moment I pledged to keep doing it for them, to find my way through. Despite all the reasons that I might feel exhausted or overwhelmed by it, I knew I had to find a way to make veterinary work for me. I will always keep on being a vet because that is exactly what I was born to do. It is a part of me, it is *who* I am, and despite the challenges and uncertainties along the way, I knew this was *not* where my own veterinary story was going to end.

RESOURCES

VetLife

VetLife is an independent charity that provides free and confidential support 24 hours a day to anyone in the UK veterinary community who is experiencing emotional, health or financial problems.

VetLife.org.uk

info@vetlife.org.uk

020 7908 6385

Samaritans

Samaritans is a unique charity dedicated to reducing feelings of isolation and disconnection that can lead to suicide, and they can be contacted day or night.

Samaritans.org

jo@samaritans.org

116 123

Pet Bereavement Support Service

The Pet Bereavement Support Service was launched in 1994 to help grieving pet owners, friends, family members and others who have contact with pet owners so that no one goes through the pain of losing a pet alone.

Bluecross.org.uk/about-pbss

pbssmail@bluecross.org.uk

0800 0966606 (8.30–20.30 every day)

Switchboard LGBT+ helpline

Switchboard provides a one-stop listening service for LGBT+ people on the phone and through Instant Messaging.

Switchboard.lgbt

0300 330 0630 (10.00–22.00 every day)

SHOUT

Shout is the UK's first and only free, confidential, 24/7 text messaging support serice for anyone who is struggling to cope.

Giveusashout.org

Text the word 'SHOUT' to 85258

ACKNOWLEDGEMENTS

With my greatest thanks.

Firstly to my agent Rosemary Scoular, and to Natalia Lucas at United Agents Ltd. This is perhaps the first time I have had the opportunity to publicly say what a great support you have both been over the past many years. Since scooping me up from the pottery floor to where we are now, your constant unwavering professionalism, gentle guidance and the occasional nudge in the right direction have once again proven to stand me in good stead – and for that, I am forever grateful.

To my commissioning editor Ru Merritt for taking a punt on this book, and on me! Then, especially huge thanks to my editor Vicky Eribo. There is simply no one else I could have done this with. Compiling this book was always going to be a rollercoaster of emotions, then midway through writing when Oliver suddenly died, things cranked up a notch! Your unequivocal compassion and understanding were so greatly appreciated. Thank you for your patience, for allowing me to write honestly and for the encouragement to keep going. I have learnt so much from you. Thank you also to Susie Bertinshaw for helping me to bring the final book together and to everyone at Seven Dials and Orion for turning this dream into a reality.

To Mark, I should apologise for hours upon hours you lost me for while I had my year-long affair with the laptop! Thank you for shouldering the tears, acting as sounding board, and for your never faltering belief. You are my rock and you mean the world to me.

Our hugest thanks to Rachael, Steve and your lovely family. Words cannot express our gratitude to you, Rachael, for the incredible gift you have given Mark and me. You have carried and carefully nurtured our little Oliver James over the months it took for me to write this book. A selfless act of generosity that will always be the greatest inspiration to us and you will forever be in our lives.

To Mum, Dad, my sister Nicola and my wider family, thank you for everything. To my dear friends Helen Henderson, Andrew Henderson, Rosie Bescoby and Sam Bescoby, for all your help with this book, your clinical brilliance and for the two decades of friendship since we met at Vet School – the hangovers, the late nights, the memories. Long may they continue! To Jay McKenny and Victoria Abbosh for your keen eye with styling and pampering for the cover shoot – for making me feel relaxed while clinging onto a chicken, surrounded by sheep and trying to encourage Oliver to stay in one place! No easy feat – but we got there, and I love you both for it. And to the brilliant Paul Stuart for all your genius-ness with the camera lens. Finally to Leanne Cornish – you are such a wonderful soul and never fail to bring joy to every situation. I absolutely could not have written this book without your constant level of encouragement, honesty and friendship.

Furthermore, I'd like to say a huge, heartfelt thank you to brilliant fellow animal enthusiast Sara Cox – from the first time we met, with me as a starstruck contestant at Middleport Pottery, to the friendship that has developed as our paths continue to cross – thank you for all your help, mentorship and support. They say never meet your idols. What utter rubbish. Thank you for everything.

A big thank you to my veterinary family at Watkins and Tasker Veterinary Surgeons. I am extremely grateful to work with such brilliant people and hold so much respect and admiration for all of you. Thank you also to all my other veterinary colleagues and peers over the years. We've shared a few laughs along the way! A heartfelt thank you also to Rosie Allister and all at Vetlife for the work and insight into veterinary mental health and the support you offer. I have learnt so much from you and on behalf of the entire profession, I want to say thank you.

Finally, to all pet owners. I feel very fortunate to have been born into a time where we can value and recognise animals as the sentient beings they are. I am always astonished and reassured by just how extraordinarily devoted people are to their pets – the care, the guardianship and the love shared. I am incredibly grateful as I could not do my job without you. Every day I rely on pet owners to spot new or unusual signs, recognise when things aren't quite right and act upon their own gut instincts to call the vet. They truly do become a part of the family and that is the greatest reflection of the love we all share for our pets.

CREDITS

Seven Dials would like to thank everyone at Orion who worked on the publication of *For the Love of Animals*.

Agent
Rosemary Scoular
United Agents Ltd

Editor
Vicky Eribo

Copy-editor
Lorraine Green

Proofreader
Sue Lascelles

Editorial Management
Susie Bertinshaw
Tierney Witty
Jane Hughes
Charlie Panayiotou
Tamara Morriss
Claire Boyle

Audio
Paul Stark
Jake Alderson
Georgina Cutler

Contracts
Dan Herron
Ellie Bowker
Alyx Hurst

Design
Nick Shah
Jessica Hart
Joanna Ridley
Helen Ewing

Picture Researcher
Nat Dawkins

Finance
Nick Gibson
Jasdip Nandra
Sue Baker
Tom Costello

Inventory
Jo Jacobs
Dan Stevens

Production
Katie Horrocks

Marketing
Brittany Sankey

Publicity
Francesca Pearce

Sales
Jen Wilson
Victoria Laws
Esther Waters
Group Sales teams across
Digital, Field, International
and Non-Trade

Operations
Group Sales Operations team

Rights
Rebecca Folland
Alice Cottrell
Ruth Blakemore
Ayesha Kinley
Marie Henckel